Adult Cochlear Implant Rehabilitation

To Nancy

With our best wishes

Anthony   Kaven   Ellen

With Compliments...

17/5/05

Dear Nancy

Very many thanks for providing a terrific forward for the book. We are all most appreciative of this + would like you to have a copy of the book from us

Best Wishes Ellen (Giles!)

CC3402

North Island
Cochlear
Implant
Programme

98 Remuera Road
Auckland 5
New Zealand
Tel: **09 520 4009**
Fax: **09 522 1622**

New Zealand

Adult Cochlear Implant Rehabilitation

Edited by

KAREN PEDLEY, BSc, MSc(AUD), MAUDSA(CCC),
Principal Audiologist, Queensland Cochlear Implant Centre,
Queensland Hearing, Arnold Janssen Centre, Brisbane Private Hospital,
Brisbane, Australia

ELLEN GILES, BA, MSc,
Senior Aural Rehabilitationist and Team Leader,
North Island Cochlear Implant Programme, National Audiology Centre,
Auckland, New Zealand

and

ANTHONY HOGAN, PhD, MARSc, QPMR,
Honorary Research Associate, Faculty of Health Sciences,
University of Sydney, Australia

W
WHURR PUBLISHERS
LONDON AND PHILADELPHIA

First Published 2005
Whurr Publishers Ltd
19b Compton Terrace, London N1 2UN, England and
325 Chestnut Street, Philadelphia PA19106, USA

British Library Cataloguing in Publication Data

A catalogue record for this book is available from the
British Library.

ISBN 1 86156 321 3

Printed and bound in the UK by Athenaeum Press Limited,
Gateshead, Tyne & Wear.

Contents

Foreword

When cochlear implantation was first becoming a viable option for adults, about twenty years ago, the common wisdom for providing aural rehabilitation could best be summarized as follows: "A clinician should do what he or she has always done—one follows the same guidelines whether providing services to someone who uses a hearing aid or whether providing services to someone who uses a cochlear implant." This one-size-fits-all approach perhaps served to reassure veteran clinicians about how to proceed, providing them with at least a starting point for how to support persons who used what were then sometimes referred to as "bionic ears."

Cochlear implants are now commonplace, used by thousands of adults worldwide, and results vary widely. Sometimes change wrought by implantation is dramatic. On the day of cochlear implant hook-up, an individual may transform from someone who is profoundly deaf to someone who can participate easily in face-to-face conversation or even use the telephone. In these instances, the experience for recipient and family members can be both exhilarating ('I can use the telephone independently!', might say a recipient and, 'I won't have to make his phone calls any more!', might say a spouse) and frightening (e.g., 'I'm going to have to start going to parties with her again?', might say the recipient and, 'He's going to start coming with my girlfriends and me to bridge club night?', might say the spouse). Sometimes, changes following cochlear implantation are realized slowly, with the cochlear implant recipient gradually learning how to use the electrical signal for speech and environmental sound recognition. Speech at first might sound odd, like talking cartoon ducks; environmental sounds may sound like alien contact—cackles and buzzes and high-pitched hums, soundtrack material for a science fiction movie. The recipient and family members may well experience discouragement, and require much encouragement to persevere until the recipient's brain adapts and sounds become meaningful. And finally, there are those heart-wrenching instances when cochlear implantation leads to unmet expectations, where the individual receives minimal benefit, no matter how long nor how diligently he or she uses the device. The recipient is disappointed, the family is disappointed.

We now know that the early approach toward aural rehabilitation is both true and not true—true in the sense that much of traditional aural rehabilitation methodology that was developed for hearing-aid users is directly applicable to cochlear implant recipients, but not true because cochlear implant recipients present unique needs and challenges, and their needs vary greatly, depending upon the success of device use. For instance, speech being a complex acoustic signal with formant regularities means that the principles of formal auditory training remain fairly standard, regardless of whether the client uses a hearing aid or a cochlear implant. On the other hand, because cochlear-implant recipients may experience rather dramatic outcomes, either positive or negative, psychosocial issues may require much more attention. The successful cochlear-implant user might need to adjust to a new self-identity and realize that he or she is now a hearing person; the unsuccessful user might have to accept life as a deaf person and manage feelings of disappointment and even despair.

This book is a masterly achievement. In an orderly and clear fashion, it covers every step of the cochlear implant process, from assessment, to "switch-on", to the traditional components of aural rehabilitation such as speech perception training, and to the less traditional topics of psychosocial support and telephone training. The authors have taken the work of many influential aural rehabilitation specialists and theoreticians and organized their methodologies and ideas into a useful, coherent structure. Perhaps even more impressive, they have expanded on tradition, and have introduced some very innovative and efficacious procedures that are uniquely suited to the needs of the very deaf and to new cochlear implant recipients. Adult Cochlear Implant Rehabilitation is an ideal text for the student who is learning about cochlear implants and an ideal reference for the practicing clinician. Aural rehabilitation has come a long way from the early days of cochlear implantation, and this book represents a stellar landmark in that evolution.

Nancy Tye Murray
Senior Research Professor
Washington University School of Medicine
St. Louis, MO USA

Preface

I was recently working with cardiologists, mapping clinical practice in the management of heart failure. During this process one of the cardiologists observed that stepping back and thinking about what one seemed to do, almost automatically as it were, was in fact quite difficult to do. Writing this book was equally difficult – like trying to explain to someone how you go about applying make-up or tying shoe laces; documenting the taken for granted is very challenging. But, in hearing rehabilitation, particularly in cochlear implants, this work desperately needed to be done.

While travelling about researching my work on psychosocial approaches to hearing rehabilitation, I had the opportunity to visit various clinics and meet with the scientists and therapists working there. When the opportunity arose I would ask them to show me their rehabilitation materials. Well, I was mostly aghast. They'd invariably pull out a jumbled file of clippings, photocopies and various other materials and say here it is! There was no apparent pedagogy in it at all – just their way of doing the work. However, working in conjunction with various rehabilitationists, it was quite obvious that they knew what they were doing and that they were highly competent at their work, although most could not readily explain to me how they actually determined where a client was up to immediately post-implant, in terms of communication skills, or why it was they chose to start a person's programme at a particular point and with certain materials, whereas for another client it would be completely different. Moreover, no one seemed to be able to say to clients succinctly, this is where we are starting from with you, this is where you'll probably end up and this is what we need to do to get you there.

These matters were of concern to me not just for the current clients, but also for the next generation of therapists coming along because new people coming into the field would have to be trained like sheepdogs on my uncle's farm! To train a new sheepdog, one would tie its collar to that of an experienced sheepdog. The trained dog would drag the trainee around as it did its work and, in time, the new dog learnt what to do. Well most of it! A lot of stress followed as the new dog finally worked out what to do when it herded the sheep unfettered. New therapists learnt implant skills by working in clinics with other therapists and picking up on what was being done. The major problem with this is that the 75% rule gets applied. Trainees tend to recall only 75% of what they are taught. Of course, in time they innovate and develop their own way of doing things, but, at the same time, subtle insights as well as specific practices taught by their predecessors can be lost. So as a group of people we thought that we could better this situation. Time will tell if the effort has been truly worth while.

The impetus behind this project was to make hearing rehabilitation with cochlear implant recipients transparent, logical and coherent. To begin with, my honours student at that time, Carolina Puleston, flew over to New Zealand to work with Ellen Giles and Merril Stewart for a few weeks. While there, Carolina conducted a file audit and worked out a basic model of the work being done. This convinced me that the goal to document a transparent and coherent process could be achieved. It would just take skill, time and effort.

The skills required to transform an idea into a reality lay in the people who have co-authored this book, particularly Karen Pedley and Ellen Giles, who contributed the bulk of talent and time into this endeavour. I am pleased to write that they are still talking to me now that the project has been successfully completed. These guys, particularly Karen, did an enormous amount of work to bring this project to a successful end. We all wondered if it would ever get finished, but thankfully it did.

My motivation for seeking to create a resource that made rehabilitation transparent and coherent was not for the purposes of producing a book or for promoting a unity of practice among therapists. Nor was it to make evident the work of therapists, as important as that is in itself, or to provide a framework for further evaluating interventions. Certainly such things may result now that these materials exist in printed form. The purpose is to enable clients to have the most effective and efficient rehabilitation experience so that their life can be all that they want it to be and more – that, as consumers of a health service, they could have programmes that have a clear beginning, a robust middle and a sensitive end. An absence of certainty creates stress. The most stressful aspect of health interventions for clients is not knowing what is happening to them, not knowing what to expect realistically and how to judge their progress objectively, and not having parameters for them to be able to say, enough is enough. Here I am reminded of the film *As Good As It Gets* with Helen Hunt and Jack Nicholson. In this movie Jack is playing the role of Mervin, a very rich man with bipolar disorder. At one point, after a crisis in his life, Jack goes to see his psychiatrist. After a slightly heated debate with his therapist he walks out of the therapist's office into a waiting room full of angst-ridden people. He stops, looks around and asks the room, *what if this is as good as it gets?* At this moment Jack is confronted with his condition and the limits of treatment, and faces the reality that he has to make the most of what he's got, to use what therapy can offer him, and in turn get on with his life, living with the residual disability that he has.

The motivation behind this book is that clients should not have to fumble their way through therapy and happen upon the realization that this is in fact as good as it gets and then suddenly just stop coming along to see us, particularly if we find it difficult to say that this is as good as it's going to get. Moreover, new colleagues coming into the field need a simpler way of developing the information and skills that they need to do their work.

Using the materials in this book you should be able to work out roughly where your client needs to start in his or her programme of rehabilitation and set goals for where he or she may end up. Such goals do not have to be set in stone. Indeed they should be revised as you go along. And as the goals are achieved and the time of plateauing approaches, we can engage with our clients in the journey of closure.

In so doing, recall that quality of life is a relative thing. When one has nothing, a little looks great. When one has a little, some looks even better. When one has some, even more would be great to have and when one has a lot, then having everything would be just fine. When we start with our clients they have little or no usable hearing. For them, things can only get better. By the time we arrive at closure with them, things have got a lot better, while at the same time we have helped them come to terms with the fact that this is as good as it will be for them and that is a fine thing, given where we have come from. We humanize this process by placing realistic boundaries around what we can offer people and by enabling them to accept and live within the boundaries unique to their condition. As the philosopher observed, we all have to make decisions in life, but mostly not in the circumstances of our choosing.

Our clients did not choose to be deafened. They did choose, however, to use implant technology. With rehabilitation we can help them make the most of the device and to move on with their lives.

Anthony Hogan

Acknowledgements

The skills, methods and ideas that we bring to this book are the outcome of many years of clinical experience, observation of colleagues, discussions with co-workers and listening to our cochlear implant patients. After over a decade of working in the field it is increasingly difficult to isolate the source of each aspect of our programme. We have endeavoured to acknowledge the sources of our ideas with the relevant chapters. In addition, we would like to thank the following people, without whom, the book would never have made it into print.

We thank the audiologists, speech pathologists and hearing therapists who read earlier drafts: Emma Rushbrooke, Sally Smith, Liza Bowen, Merril Stewart, Elena DeAmbrosis, Dimity Dornan, Dr. Stizanne Purdy and Christopher Lind.

Thanks go to Professor Brian Hardaker who gave Karen the benefit of his academic writing experience, Professor Bruce Black for comments on medical aspects and Michael Condon for many helpful discussions on the psychological perspective.

Thanks to Merren Davies and Simon Melville at Cochlear Ltd, Cassandra Brown and Ilona Anderson at MED-EL and Ryoko Imai at Advanced Bionics for supplying technical information and photographs.

Thanks also to Geoff Plant for discussions about rehabilitation methods and setting such a wonderful example of dedicated and self-less work. His International Aural Rehabilitation conferences in Portland, Maine, have provided a valuable opportunity to share ideas and inspirations with other rehabilitationists working with adults.

We thank Denzil Brooks, Nancy Tye Murray and Mary Mitchell for inspiring Karen's and Ellen's interest in aural rehabilitation and providing early mentoring.

Thank you to our patients who have enthusiastically entered into our CI rehabilitation programmes and for the feedback they have provided over the years on our rehabilitation methods and materials.

And not least, a huge thank you to Karen and Ellen's wonderfully supportive husbands and respective families who put up with our endless absences while working on the book and read endless drafts. Thanks too to Anthony's Karen for staying with yet another project.

Contributors

Lisa Dyer, BAppSc(SPPATH), CertCounsPsych, MSPAA, Speech Pathologist, Child and Adolescent Mental Health Service, Southern Health, Dandenong, Australia

Ellen Giles, BA, MSc, Senior Aural Rehabilitationist and Team Leader, North Island Cochlear Implant Programme, National Audiology Centre, Auckland, New Zealand

Susan Hamrouge, MSc, RegMRCSLT, Speech and Language Therapist/Audiologist, Specialist Support Service, Flash Ley Resource Centre, Stafford, UK

Anthony Hogan, PhD, MARSC, QPMR, Partner, Healthcare, Blue Moon Research and Planning in Sydney and Honorary Research Fellow, Faculty of Health Sciences, University of Sydney, Australia

Christopher Lind, BA, BAppsc(spPath), DipAud, MAppSc, MSPAA, MAudSA(CCC), Lecturer in Audiology, Department of Speech Pathology and Audiology, Flinders University, Adelaide, Australia

Andrea Lynch, BSpThy, MSocSci (Counselling), MQCA, Rehabilitation Consultant/Speech Pathologist/Counsellor, Hill End, Australia

Karen Pedley, BSc, MSc(Aud), MAudSA(CCC), Principal Audiologist, Queensland Cochlear Implant Centre, Queensland Hearing, Arnold Janssen Centre, Brisbane Private Hospital, Brisbane, Australia

Sarah Worsfold, BSocSci, Dip RCSLT, MCSLT, Reg HPC, Research Speech and Language Therapist, Hearing Outcomes Project, Child Health Department, Southampton General Hospital, Southampton, UK

Chapter 1
Introduction: towards a more holistic and transdisciplinary model of rehabilitation

ANTHONY HOGAN

> The waters we leaped into are not just deep, but uncharted. We are not even at the crossroads: for crossroads to be crossroads, there must be first roads. Now we know that we *make* roads - the only roads there are and can be - and we do this solely by *walking* them.
>
> Bauman (1995)

Shirley Ackehurst documented her experience of having a cochlear implant in a book entitled *Broken Silence* (1989). In this book, Shirley presents her experience of having an implant as miraculous. There is little doubt that the results of the implant process are life changing. However, the reality for many clients is that communication skills come from the hard yards that they, their therapist and their family put into the rehabilitation process. This is mostly hidden work. Rarely are TV film crews called in to tape yet another mapping session, or to capture someone doing yet another tracking exercise, sometimes getting it right, sometimes getting it wrong. Although this hard rehabilitation work may lack the glamour of the switch-on day, the practised clinician knows just how essential it is to a client's successful outcome. The miracle metaphor does, however, capture one reality - that each person's surgical outcome is unique, that, as the client's clinician, we have the task of working out where he or she is with the device, and in turn, subsequently to plan a path forward, where the individual can come to maximize what the device can offer him or her. When I first became involved in implant work, more than 10 years ago, a systematic literature on how to manage this process was not available. Certainly there were competent clinicians practising in various clinics; their skills base had been developed over many years of clinical work. They inherently knew what to do with their clients: where to start with them, what to work on and to what ends. Moreover, they knew when the client's needs fell outside their area of expertise, recognizing the need to call in another person, often from a different professional background, to help the client through a specific need or challenge. Implicitly, these clinicians developed what we are now referring to as a holistic model of rehabilitation within an implant programme.

The importance of providing clients with a well-structured holistic programme of rehabilitation has not always been recognized by clinics. Some have believed that adult outcomes result simply from mapping the device and leaving clients to make of it what they will. Clients, unsurprisingly, have their own thoughts on such a process, e.g. Jack is a health professional who received an implant from such a programme. For him, the clinic's excitement about the technology completely exceeded his experience of the switch-on process, which was, in his terms, a disappointment:

> So umm, all the electrodes work. They say 'fine!' see. So they put the program processor and turn it on and expecting me to be delighted, and this is [not] different from other people, I've compared. What I heard was nothing like normal sound at all, it was just like birds twittering. It was all high-pitched non-sense. I was dismayed. I thought how can I make any sense of that?

Jack's professional assessment of his own needs was that he required post-switch-on rehabilitation, yet his clinic did not provide such assistance. So Jack imposed on himself a rigorous training programme, including attempting to learn a foreign language, based on listening to audio-inputs. He also tried to learn a new musical instrument. Through regular listening, learning and practice with systems that enhanced the demands of the brain to discriminate sounds, Jack developed a rehabilitation programme that he hoped would yield the outcomes that he desired.

Most of our clients do not have Jack's high level of graduate professional training or the conceptual abilities to be able to develop for themselves a coherent rehabilitation programme. Moreover, they should not have to work out their own programme or manage it on their own. Indeed, as a group of professionals we found it a challenge to bring these materials together. How can we realistically expect our clients to be able to do this on their own?

Of course, situations like Jack's require a highly competent client, an uncomplicated implant process and a client with a psychologically well-adjusted disposition. Many clinical experiences with clients fail to meet one of these criteria. People are complicated beings and problems with the implant itself can have little to do with the issue of client adjustment. Rick observes:

I find the only thing I've got against it, is the clarity. The clarity like as far as anything else is concerned, like I can hear a plane, took me a long time to figure it out what the noise was, but I can hear a plane going over the home. Ah, but that sort of thing I could never hear before. I sit there, I couldn't hear the telephone ring. If I got this on [speech processor] I hear the telephone ring. I know the telephone's ringing. Like doors slamming. It takes a long time to pick up what it is to sort of balance what's going on. That takes a long time. But, I don't think like in meself that I've got any real complaints about it. Um . . . I mean to say it's just a disappointment. Not a complaint. You know what – it's a disappointment, I wouldn't complain about it. Like [they] just asked me once did I just want to leave it [the speech processor] there – you know and forget about it. But I thought oh well, I keep it going.

As far as Rick is concerned, the implant sounds like chipmunks. It provides him with an environmental input and assists lip-reading. He is disappointed with the outcome. It is nothing like the sensation of sound as he remembers it. In the drama laid out by Rick several simultaneous processes are in place. First, after implantation, unresolved personal factors arose that flavoured Rick's views on his implant outcome. In post-implant counselling it became apparent that Rick was motivated by guilt to come into the implant programme after reading about the implant in the media. He had felt guilty about the burden that his deafness has imposed on his wife for all these years. He wanted to do whatever he could to reduce this burden; he felt that this was his responsibility. He underwent surgery and began using a cochlear implant. He was dismayed by the sound, by the fact that he still had to lip-read. He then reflected on a transitional moment, the moment when he contemplated giving up the speech processor, leaving it in the clinic and going home. It was another moment of failure and he was disappointed in himself and the programme. Ironically, the programme deemed him to be a great success because he performed very well on speech and listening evaluation tests.

Like Jack's programme, Rick's clinic did not usually provide pre- or post-implant counselling. It was inevitable then, given Rick's essential motivations, that, irrespective of the technical outcome, he would face significant problems adjusting to his implant. The solution that he sought was to an emotional, not an auditory, problem. Unfortunately, a lot of clinical time was wasted on Rick because his needs had not been accurately identified or managed. Part of Rick's difficulties occurred because a coherent, holistic and competency-based assessment and rehabilitation programme was not in place. The clinician knew that Rick's problems fell outside technical areas, but lacked the tools to demonstrate this to him.

We set out to develop this text so that clinicians could have access to a range of practical materials that would enable them readily to assess where a client is with regard to progress with an implant and, in turn, to provide the client with a quality rehabilitation programme and experience. As practitioners we recognized that we used specific strategies to assess where a client was and, in turn, to design and implement an intervention that would meet his or her communicative and psychosocial needs. We also recognized that within this was an implicit philosophy of competency-based training and a firm professional commitment to the vital role that rehabilitation plays in achieving optimal clinical outcomes. An individual needs to master certain things before other abilities will develop. The biggest challenge for us was to document what we did so that others could have the benefit of it. And so this text was born.

We refer to this overall process as a holistic model of rehabilitation. In a holistic model of rehabilitation, Rick would have undergone counselling concerning his feelings of guilt, helping him and his wife work through their desire for an implant versus their wish to reaffirm their relationship in all its difficulties. Jack would not have had to work out his own auditory training programme – one would have been tailored to meet his needs. To arrive at this model of work, we had to stand back and ask ourselves, what is the purpose of a cochlear implant programme? In posing this question to ourselves we recognized that the objectives of implant programmes have changed over the years, as the technology has developed. In the early days of the programme, achieving a sense of sound was an optimal outcome. Enabling a person to communicate through hearing and speech has become more real as the technology developed. These days we are now focusing on quality of life, employment and relational outcomes. Who knows what will come next!

This rapidly changing environment has posed considerable challenges to staff providing implant rehabilitation. Implicitly, expectations for what the clinician could achieve have changed, but rehabilitation materials and resources have not kept up. In consequence, each clinician has grappled to develop materials that will work for their client. Few have had time to step back and reflect on the need for a structured approach to rehabilitation, even if they have in fact been practising it themselves. As well, each clinician has often only had her own background of training and the limited resources of her clinic to draw on.

Our approach to rehabilitation resulted from the unique circumstances of life that brought us together, as seemingly isolated rehabilitation professionals, who realized that together we could offer our clients more than if we proceeded alone. Coupled with our deep mutual respect for the skills set that each of us possessed was the realization that all of us could make an important contribution to the lives of our clients. For us, quality rehabilitation was something more than a matter of chance. It required having well-trained professionals available, in sufficient numbers and with sufficient time, to provide the new cochlear implant recipient with the training and support that they required in order to be able to maximize what the device could offer them. Initially we were unique individuals who had developed expert skills in rehabilitation over a long period of time and who had come to drive the orientation of our own programmes. Our professional backgrounds included audiology but also speech and language therapy, hearing therapy and counselling. As we came to work together, we formed a professional melting pot of transdisciplinary work, which produced a rich blend of therapeutic strategies. I say transdisciplinary rather than interdisciplinary because, within a transdisciplinary approach, not only do we learn from each other, but we also all learn to do parts of each other's role, whereas in interdisciplinary work strict professional boundaries remain – and where strict boundaries exist, petty jealousies form and divisions arise.

The success of our transdisciplinary work also stemmed from the recognition of the unique contribution that each of us individually, and as a team, could make to people's lives. It was as a result of working in this interactive fashion that the need for this book became quite apparent, because so much of what we were doing was unique, or had been uniquely developed from the original work of others, it needed to be written down so that others could learn it, and learn it properly. We wanted to be able to do the work that we saw our colleagues doing. Moreover, as we were often geographically isolated from each other, we needed to be able to transport the skills set back to our own centres and to complete the skills transfer process accurately and faithfully. Further, we saw the need for people coming into implant work in the future to have the opportunity to access a range of materials rather than having either to reinvent the wheel or to try to develop the skills set from someone else and perhaps, in so doing, miss out on essential parts of it.

Most importantly, we remained deeply aware that our clients often had goals that were different to those of people who were running a *programme*. Transdisciplinary work implicitly includes the client within the structure of the service delivery model. Certainly we knew that our clients wanted to be able to hear, but moreover they sought to get back the life that they lost before deafness. Clients do not relate well to the idea of achieving a percentage improvement on a word score. It is a fairly abstract and meaningless exercise that is disconnected from the world that they seek to reattain:

> I think it would be marvellous [pauses] just to have the opportunity of talk with people in a really in-depth way and being helped to draw out your own thoughts. Oh that would be wonderful. That's what I lost. [Carol]

This implicit client goal of effective, interactive communication sets up a great contradiction for the implant as an intervention. Because, on the one hand, this is exactly what is intended – to restore hearing so that people can get back on with their lives. But, at the same time, it is very unlikely that this will be the complete outcome. First, it is likely that a level of impaired hearing will remain. Second, because of the various experiences that the person has gone through, the person he or she knew, as him- or herself, has changed forever. As the outcomes of the process become apparent, a central part of the clinical role is to enable the client to see that the outcome *is* the outcome. Is it not unethical to lead a client to believe that things will get better (and in the client's eyes this can still be taken to mean that things will significantly improve) when they will not really, or only marginally? Is it right continually to tell clients that they are doing *really* well, when in fact they are not? At what point do we enable clients to acknowledge that something in addition to the implant is required in order for them to achieve fulfilling communication. When we arrive at this point, what do we do? It is certainly possible to avoid discussing these things. Indeed many clients realize in themselves that it is pointless persisting with certain therapies any more and they simply stop coming to clinic. An unspoken deal is struck between the clinic and the patient, resulting in a stalemate. Both know that the result is not what it could be, but to confront that reality is to go into uncharted territory that may well be feared.

The move into a more formalized psychosocial phase of therapy serves as a right of passage for both the client and his or her key therapist. It signals for both that the time for looking to the implant for further gains has come to an end and it is time to move on to other things. Of course, it would be naïve to see the psychosocial process as a panacea for all unresolved issues in implant work. The psychosocial process should serve to enable the person to engage with the idea that, with the technology, *this is as good as it gets*, and that in turn one must now adapt one's sense of self and one's behaviour to a new way of living. It engages people in an adjustment process but it does not necessarily enable people to resolve their issues. Just as with any grief and identity change process, these things take months and years to work through. What is important is that people first begin to look beyond the technology for answers to their problems, and second that there is support available to the client as they work through this process – support in terms of an empathetic ear but also in terms of psychotherapy where it is needed.

It is the desire to regain what has been lost that first drives the rehabilitative effort and which is also at the heart of the emotionally challenging times that result. A brief scan across the pages of this book highlights the fact that not only is there hard, skills-based work ahead, but that the terrain of rehabilitation is marked with many emotional and psychological challenges. Moments of shear stress, worry, panic, frustration, boredom and elation move in and out of people's lives as they (re)learn to hear and live again. We promote a holistic approach to rehabilitation because it is plainly evident that an implant programme is not just about technology; it is not just about fancy therapeutic techniques or strategies. It is about working with people in their daily struggles to achieve important goals. We recognize that, on the road to the future, there will be tough days when all our science lets us down and lets the clients down. Not to recognize this is to deny the humanity and frailness of the people with whom we are working and to steam-roller over their needs and feelings.

So, as you scan the pages of this book, you will see a refined clinical sensitivity that offers insight into the impact that the process of going through an implant intervention has on the client. You will find insights as to how to adapt your practice, to take these needs into account. It is as simple and as complex as this. How well I recall a woman relating to me the essential stress of learning to use her implant. Day in and day out she would progress through mapping sessions that she found very stressful, yet the clinic was completely unaware of the stress that she was under. It would only be after she left the clinic following her mapping sessions that she would break down and cry alone. What a difference even a simple question such as 'how are you finding this today?' may have made to her rehabilitation experience.

For each client, rehabilitation is a journey. Some will start in adjustment programmes such as the Link Centre in Eastbourne (England) and will develop communication skills without technologies such as an implant. Others will start with an implant and then build on their communicative skills set. Either way, clients and clinicians will have to put in the time to enable the client to re-take the place in the world that deafness took from him or her. The detail of this text is a recognition of the hidden work, pain, effort and struggle undertaken by so many people in enabling someone to resume his or her life more fully, in the hearing world.

There are several ways to use this text. First, it is laid out in a fashion that follows the seemingly logical flow of the implant process. From an educational point of view, systematically working through the text chapter by chapter is the way to go. Second, we have tried to write a text that is, as the title suggests, a clinician's handbook. To this end, the text can be laid out on a desk or in the therapy room, at a given exercise. We have found that many of our co-clinicians have found this a useful way to work on exercises with clients, with the materials in front of you as a resource.

References

Ackehurst S (1989) Broken Silence. Sydney: Collins
Bauman Z (1995) Life in Fragments: Essays in postmodern morality. Oxford: Blackwell

Chapter 2
The assessment of adult cochlear implant candidates

KAREN PEDLEY AND ELLEN GILES

The assessment of cochlear implant candidates is an important component of a cochlear implant programme. Crucial decisions are made about the patient's hearing management and, hence, the future quality of life of the patient and those close to him or her. A coordinated, structured, holistic, comprehensive approach, beginning with the patient's communication goals, is advocated, because it has been found by the authors to produce good outcomes. The emphasis is on finding a workable and effective management plan for the patient's severe hearing problems, rather than 'to implant or not to implant'. The patient is fully and accurately informed and supported at all stages, enabling full participation in the decision process and, hence, greater commitment to the final decision at the end of the assessment period.

This chapter focuses on the non-medical components of candidacy assessment, with emphasis on the management of patient and family preoperative expectations. The postoperative satisfaction with the device, and whether cochlear implantation is judged as 'successful' by all those involved, hangs on managing this crucial aspect of pre-implant assessment well. A variety of approaches currently in use is described so that clinicians and therapists can incorporate into their own practice those most suitable to their patient population, their resources and the professional skills that they have available. The formal components of the assessment aim to establish whether the patient is a suitable candidate from medical, audiological, rehabilitation and psychological perspectives.

The chapter is divided into seven sections. The first provides an overview of cochlear implant assessment procedures and the environment in which they take place. The second discusses the information exchange during the patient's initial contact with the clinic. In the third, the audiological and otolaryngological assessment is described and in the fourth, rehabilitation assessment, issues of communication needs and psychological assessment are discussed. In the fifth section, different ways of managing the expectations of the patient and their family are discussed. The sixth covers the practical issues that require information counselling, and in the seventh we describe how the information is brought together to decide on an appropriate course of action.

Introduction to cochlear implantation

What is a cochlear implant and what can it do?

A cochlear implant (CI) is a device that has become an important management option for severe-to-profoundly deaf individuals who derive insufficient benefit from hearing aids (Figure 2.1). A CI consists of a microphone, which collects the acoustic information, an external processor, which analyses the incoming signal, an internal processor and an electrode array, which is surgically placed inside the cochlea. The speech processor converts the acoustic sound signal into an electrical signal. The electrical stimulation of the electrode array replaces the transduction process that is performed by the sensory cells of the inner ear in the normal cochlea. In this way the CI provides direct input to the central auditory pathways by electrically stimulating the spiral ganglion cells of the auditory nerve.

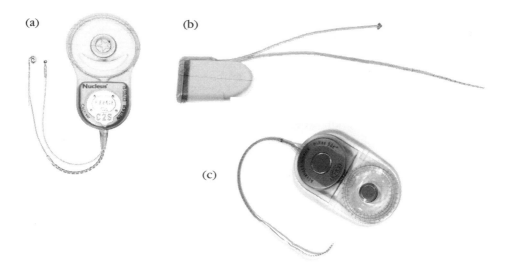

Figure 2.1 The cochlear implants produced by the three main manufacturers: (a) Nucleus CI24 (contour advanced); (b) MED-EL Combi 40+; and (c) Advanced Bionics HiRes 90K Bionic Ear Implant. (Photographs kindly supplied courtesy of Cochlear Ltd, MED-EL and Advanced Bionics Corp., respectively.)

The technology of the modern CI has enabled many CI recipients to perceive and recognize environmental sounds and to reach near-normal word comprehension in quiet situations. With the addition of lip-reading, many CI users are able to hold a conversation with a familiar speaker with ease. Some CI recipients learn to enjoy music through the implant. However, individuals are still likely to experience difficulty hearing in group situations and in background noise. Hearing over the telephone is now possible for an increasing number of CI recipients.

A number of patient-related factors appear to be important as possible predictors of cochlear implant performance, including duration of deafness, age at onset, length of *profound* deafness, amount of residual hearing and preoperative hearing aid use (Gantz et al., 1988; Parkin et al., 1989; Shipp and Nedzelski, 1995; Blamey et al., 1996; Kawashima et al., 1998; Van Dijk, et al., 1999). Although the factors provide helpful guidelines for counselling, clinicians must be careful about making clinical generalizations and the trends should not be used to exclude patients. It has been estimated that these factors account for only around 50% of the variability in outcomes, making it difficult to provide the patient with more than a general indication of likely outcome. Clinicians must therefore supplement published trends with the experience reported by patients using current devices to portray a realistic picture for each individual. It is a skill in itself to achieve the right balance in expectation counselling and ensure that the message has been understood – to be sufficiently conservative so that expectations remain realistic while emphasizing the possible positive benefits.

The cochlear implant team

In a multidisciplinary team each member brings a different perspective and different skills to the programme. A CI team typically includes surgeons, audiologists and rehabilitationists. The role of rehabilitationist may be taken by speech and language therapists, audiologists or, in countries such as the UK, hearing therapists. Increasingly, cochlear implant teams include a psychologist and this role is discussed in detail later in the chapter under 'Rehabilitation assessment' pp 26–30. In some programmes, a social worker or counsellor may undertake some of the psychologist's function.

Identification of CI candidates

The assessment process begins when a patient presents to either the implant clinic or local audiological and/or otolaryngological professionals. Basic audiological assessment (pure-tone, speech and immitance audiometry) may be performed that shows a severe-to-profound hearing loss or greater, and the patient reports minimal benefit from hearing aids and other assistive devices but has a desire to be part of the hearing world. Where distance from the implant clinic makes this more practical, local professionals may also perform components of the candidacy assessment (see below). Each cochlear implant clinic will have its own audiological indications for acceptance of referrals. The three most commonly used measures are unaided pure-tone thresholds, aided thresholds (which reflect the hearing aid wearer's ability to detect all sounds in speech at normal conversational levels) and measures of functional hearing such as aided open-set speech recognition. In some clinics the age of onset of profound deafness may be a criterion. In the authors' clinics, adults with congenital profound hearing losses are not excluded because the benefits of environmental sound awareness and the use of the implant sound as an aid to speech reading, for example, are considered as valid as the open-set speech recognition scores obtained by postlingually deafened adults (Rushbrooke and Pedley, 2002), e.g. the current Cochlear Ltd indications for referral to an implant centre are:

- Unaided thresholds are, at best, moderate to severe in the low to mid frequencies and severe to profound in the mid to high frequencies.
- Aided thresholds in one or more frequencies greater than 55 dBSPL (sound pressure level).
- Less than 60% in either ear on individual ear, open-set pre-recorded sentences presented at 65 dBSPL.

Certainly, the depth and breadth of assessment required to make an informed decision make CI candidacy one of the most time-consuming processes in the field of audiology. This is appropriate because cochlear implantation is elective surgery, involving sophisticated implanted and high-cost devices, and requires (initially intensive) life-long management.

Overview of the components of assessment

The assessment process detailed in Figure 2.2 illustrates the essential components and recommended sequence of a candidate assessment. It is designed to identify unsuitable candidates as early as possible in the assessment procedure, so that only those patients who meet the audiological criteria (either the centre's own or those recommended by the implant manufacturer) are subjected to the more costly and invasive procedures. A coordinated, flexible team approach ensures that the programme meets the patient's needs. The need for several appointments with different professionals over a period of time is not disadvantageous. It allows the patient and family time to assimilate the information, discuss it with their

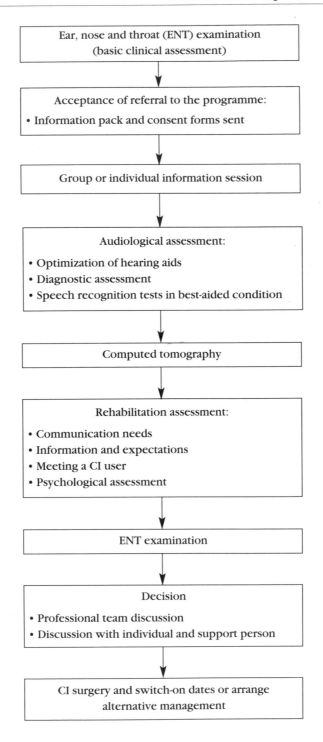

Figure 2.2 The components of a cochlear implant (CI) assessment.

support network, prepare new questions and hear different viewpoints. Profoundly deaf patients usually appreciate avoiding lengthy appointments and too many assessments on one day because communication is very tiring. When all of the assessments are complete, the CI team meets to discuss the results and impressions of the patient. Factors that may impact on post-implant management are discussed. If the patient is not a candidate, an alternative management scheme may be proposed. The recommendations of the team are then discussed in detail with the patient and family.

Beginning the assessment process

First contact

A patient may be more comfortable with a clinic if the first contact conveys an impression of a team dedicated to solving his or her communication problems rather than one focused on medical procedures. Clinicians should not underestimate the importance of a sensitive approach to the patient's first visit to the clinic. Many patients have attended several appointments with local professionals to obtain a referral to the CI programme and may be feeling this is the 'last hope' of obtaining an improvement in hearing status. The patient now has to meet the team of people who will (in their eyes, at least) decide the future management of their hearing. The emotional energy expended by the patient in anticipation of this appointment may be likened to attending an important job interview, and many patients are very anxious on arrival and as a result tire quickly, both of which are factors that impact on their communication ability. The patient's concerns may include whether the team members are friendly, patient, empathetic, approachable and easy to communicate with. This is understandable because many will be accustomed to people talking to their partners rather than to them directly, and to displays of impatience. Other concerns at this first visit include 'will it work for me?', 'will it be worth all this effort?' and even 'will I say all the right things to make sure I get accepted?'. Some patients have described the assessment process as an obstacle course in which they have to overcome all the hurdles. Making sure that patients understand why all the appointments are necessary and focusing on the desire to find solutions are important.

An information pack is one way to convey the clinic's approach to auditory rehabilitation. Of particular interest to novice implant candidates are manufacturer's booklets describing the implant, testimonials from CI recipients, information about the assessment process, particularly why so many tests are necessary, and the clinic's postoperative rehabilitation programme. Inclusion of a typical appointment schedule prepares the patient for the time-consuming nature of the assessment process and the commitment required. Some clinics use in-house information booklets to introduce patients to all of the potential solutions to the hearing problems and how these may be accessed. This holistic approach encourages the patient to make a choice, rather than considering other options only if they find an implant inappropriate.

A patient questionnaire can be a valuable tool at this stage. It can save the CI clinicians' time by providing an overall profile of each patient, identifying the important issues and any special needs. Clinicians with experience in taking history details from profoundly hearing-impaired patients will appreciate the value of written information – the clinician can focus on the patient, providing an opportunity for reflective listening and observation of communication patterns. It can be useful to ask questions about the patient's general health, hearing history and current degree of handicap, hearing devices used, hearing abilities in different situations, coping strategies, additional needs and knowledge about cochlear implants. Such questions encourage patients to take a step back and examine their current communication methods and the impact of their hearing loss. This can help them to verbalize their needs when meeting members of the implant team. Some clinics may use the questionnaire to prioritize the most needy patients. An example of such a questionnaire appears in Appendix 1.

The support person

Many clinics encourage each patient to involve a support person from the outset. The support person plays an important role in providing emotional support, encouraging the patient, liaising with the clinic in appointment scheduling, providing background information and often providing transport. Ideally, this person will provide support throughout the assessment period, at switch-on and during the important first 3 months post-implant as a practice partner for auditory training, conversation practice and providing feedback to the rehabilitationist.

In most cases, the support person would be a partner, family friend or relation. When a patient does not have a support person, some clinics offer to provide one. This could be a CI user, hearing-aid user or volunteer involved with the clinic. The benefits of involving a support person, in the opinion of the authors, far outweigh any disadvantages, and are detailed below:

- Patients need someone with whom they can discuss their hopes and their doubts. It is important that this person is accurately informed.
- The support person is less likely to be stressed and hence less likely to misinterpret information.
- Any myths, unrealistic expectations or misunderstandings on the part of the support person can be addressed directly in the discussion process.

- The support person can provide a vital information link for extended family and friends, conveying information about what a CI can and cannot do.
- When the support person attends the clinic, the family relationships and dynamics can be observed. Changes that may be brought about by the implant can be identified and discussed. This is important for providing ongoing support and for the long-term success of the intervention.

Being aware of the potential pitfalls will enable the CI team to maximize the benefit of the support person. These include:

- A partner may not be supportive of implantation and this may sabotage the process. The CI team would wish to discuss these issues openly with all concerned so that negative opinions are identified early on in the assessment process.
- The partner may not respect the patient's choice. In some cases, partners develop a dominant role and become the 'voice' for the patient in decision-making. Some partners may be reluctant to give up that role.
- The patients may prefer to be independent in seeking out this form of help for themselves, and may not wish to have a support person 'placed' with them. In this case, rather than merely respecting the patient's preference, the team should explore the patient's motives for this independence.

Informing patients: group sessions or individual counselling?

Information sessions provide the candidate with information about the device and pre- and post-implant management. Suggestions for format and content are given below. The session is of most benefit early in the assessment process because, once informed, a patient may decide that he or she does not wish to pursue a management option involving surgery, or visits to an implant clinic for the rest of his or her life, for example. The information may be offered on a one-on-one basis or in a group format. Both have advantages. The one-on-one approach enables more focused management of patients with special needs or additional handicaps. The group approach can save a considerable amount of time for clinics implanting large numbers of patients. In both formats the support person is included for the reasons previously described.

The comparative effectiveness of group sessions versus individual information counselling has not been subjected to formal scientific assessment. However, the benefits reported by patients attending the New Zealand programme in Auckland include:

- Reduced feelings of isolation: meeting others with severe hearing difficulties, patients and their support people realize that they are not the only person in this situation. Some patients go on to form friendships that provide mutual support through the assessment process.
- The opportunity to become acquainted with team members in an informal environment.
- Greater ease of assimilation of information in the relaxed environment where they are not the sole focus of attention.
- The interactive, facilitated nature of the session was reported to be an effective way to learn.
- Patients reported that in a small group they felt more comfortable asking questions that they perceived to be very basic.
- Listening to the concerns, questions and discussions initiated by other participants.

For the clinicians, a group session provides an opportunity to observe the patient in an interactive environment, to assess the communication skills informally and the relationship with the support person, and to observe any special needs that should be considered at future sessions.

Practical considerations in running a group session

The organizer should consider patient numbers, the environment, aids to communication and presentation style. Limiting numbers to three patients, each with a support partner, promotes easier communication and greater interaction between group members. More than this number could make the listening task too difficult for severely deafened adults. Facilitation is more effective with two clinicians, such as an audiologist and a rehabilitationist, whose combined knowledge and skills enable them to field a variety of questions.

If a choice of rooms is available, the clinician should be mindful that reduced reverberation and good lighting (so that shadows are not cast over any participants' faces) assist speech comprehension and lip-reading, respectively. Seating arrangements that enable all participants, including the clinicians, to be positioned around the same table can facilitate communication. Enhanced visibility and proximity of participants is important, because lip-reading and hearing for hearing-impaired participants become increasingly difficult at distances greater than 1–1.5 m. This also has implications for group size.

Name badges for all participants (clearly written in at least font size 26 so that it can be read across a table) help to 'break the ice', enable people to feel part of the group and facilitate the introduction process, because hearing and lip-reading names is often difficult. A sound field amplification system, FM system or signing interpreter may be required to facilitate communication for all participants. Individual requirements and equipment needs of group members should be checked with participants in advance of the meeting. A session agenda can assist the hearing-impaired participants to follow the discussion. If the discussion moves away from the agenda, this should be made clear to participants because people with a severe or profound hearing loss are likely to miss a change in subject and are unlikely to ask for clarification. Questions should be encouraged and clarifications made at the end of each topic, before moving on to a new subject.

Feedback from our patients is that an informal presentation works well, with laminated visual aids and graphs that can be passed around. The facilitator should bear in mind that a severely hearing-impaired listener may benefit from short breaks to prevent eye strain and fatigue. Individual information folders containing spare notepaper, pens and copies of the information from the presentation enable patients to concentrate on, and participate in, the discussion. The folder can include sources of further information about cochlear implants (e.g. website addresses for the CI manufacturers, CI forums, local support groups and references to books written by CI users).

Suggested group session format

A group information session of 1.5 hours may take the following format:

- Introduction and welcome: 'welcome' message on a board helps to set the 'tone' of the session, introduce the clinicians and create a relaxed and non-threatening environment.
- Some guidelines to enhance communication may be presented, e.g. one speaker at a time. Any participant's 'right to pass' should be respected.
- Clinicians invite participants to introduce themselves and say a few words about their hearing situation. Support partners are encouraged to add any additional information that they feel would be helpful.
- The clinician or facilitator presents a brief overview of the session and checks with group members that the content addresses all of their issues and concerns. This allows for the needs of the whole group.
- The components of the cochlear implant candidate assessment process are described.
- Implant candidacy and likely outcomes with the device (see below) are discussed.
- The implant device(s), speech processors and how they are worn are demonstrated.

- Basic information about duration of surgery and hospital stay is provided.
- An overview is given of the long-term commitment required for post-implant mapping and rehabilitation to maximize communication potential and post-implant care. This is especially important when either the patient or the support person is working and for those living some distance from the clinic.
- The value of a support network and the role of the support person are discussed.
- Towards the end of the session a few minutes can be set aside for the clinicians to work individually with each patient and support partner to discuss any immediate concerns.

Frequently asked questions at group information sessions

Clinicians should anticipate and be able to answer a range of questions. These are likely to include the following areas:

- Sound quality from the implant and the time taken for this to improve
- Outcomes in specific situations and outcome predictors
- Individual variation
- Success and failure rate
- Issues of equipment maintenance and the technical support provided by the programme.

Sound quality with a cochlear implant

The point to stress here is that the quality of sound with a CI at initial fitting may be rather poor and unlike anything that they have heard before. Some people describe sound as being 'harsh' and others as 'squeaky' or 'high-pitched'. Patients should realize that the sound quality may take a few weeks or even months to become more natural sounding for speech and environmental sounds. The importance of being patient and persevering with the use of the CI, even when the sound quality is not at its best, can be discussed. A brief illustrated overview of the speech-processing strategies available may be of interest to some groups.

In our experience, the patient's understanding about the probable sound quality from an implant is enhanced by inviting an articulate experienced CI recipient to give a first-hand account of his or her own experiences. However, a further opportunity to meet with a CI user on a one-on-one basis is also recommended. This is discussed below.

Outcomes for hearing in specific situations

Patients do not understand the jargon that clinicians use to express speech perception scores. Outcomes should relate to everyday situations, such as whether they will be able to communicate with their partner, hear the grandchildren, enjoy TV, use the phone, hear in a meeting or hold down a job.

Clinicians may find it helpful to present this information by using patient outcome data to illustrate the range of outcomes. Graphs from the New Zealand Cochlear Implant Programme illustrate this point (Figure 2.3). Graphs may be used to show the number of CI users on the programme able to use the telephone, for example, or the extent to which CI users continue to rely on visual clues.

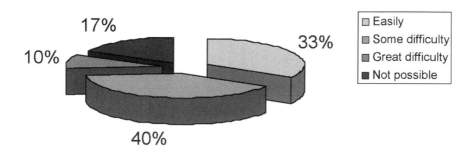

Figure 2.3 Outcomes for hearing with a cochlear implant in specific situations: able to have a two-way conversation on the telephone with family and friends (*n* = 63). (Data from Audit of New Zealand (Adult) CI Programme (2000).)

In discussing indicators of outcome it is best to present general outcomes based on specific factors. These include onset of the hearing loss (pre-, peri- or postlingual), duration and course of the hearing loss (e.g. outcomes for those with a recent hearing loss versus those with a longstanding/gradually progressing loss) and prior hearing aid use (i.e. prolonged period of auditory deprivation versus continued use of hearing aid).

Individual variation

Some patients find it reassuring to see the variation in rate of improvement for different CI users on speech perception, hearing ability and other measures. Typical case studies could show the progress for individuals in understanding words in sentences, recognizing environmental sounds, monitoring their own voice and understanding group conversation, as well as abilities rated by the support person such as ease of communication with the CI recipient. Graphs showing individual scores preoperatively and post switch-on and typical progress from switch-on, through 1 month, 3 months, 6 months and 9 months after the switch-on, may be useful. Examples are shown in Figures 2.4 and 2.5.

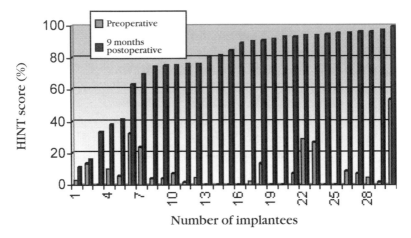

Figure 2.4 Comparison of preoperative and 9 months after switch-on scores for CI24 users ($n = 30$). (Data from New Zealand (Adult) CI Programme (2000).)

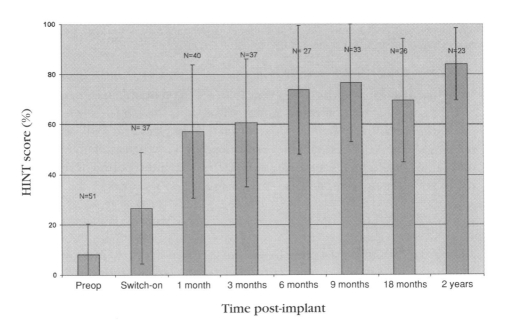

Figure 2.5 Improvement over time for CI24 users on hearing in noise test (HINT) sentences. (Data from New Zealand (Adult) CI Programme (2000).)

Success and failure rate

Patients are mainly interested in the likelihood of device failure and interdevice comparisons where relevant. This information is available in regular updates from the manufacturers. Patients may also ask whether any CI recipients on the programme have required re-implantation as a result of device failure.

Equipment maintenance and technical support

The key point to cover here is that speech processors, like hearing aids, are delicate electrical instruments that need to be kept clean and dry. Patients should have a broad idea of battery consumption and costs of batteries and spare parts. They will be particularly interested in the local availability of devices on loan in the event of breakdown.

Audiological assessment

Both the patient's local audiologist and the CI team audiologist may contribute to the audiological assessment. The aims of the audiological assessment are (1) to confirm the degree of hearing loss at frequencies important for speech perception, (2) to identify any factors that may affect the relative suitability of each ear for cochlear implantation, (3) to confirm the presence of a functioning auditory nerve, (4) to identify those patients with an auditory disorder not compatible with cochlear implantation and (5) to establish whether the patient meets various audiological criteria for implantation. The audiological criteria address the degree of hearing loss and the patient's aided speech-recognition ability. The content of the diagnostic audiological assessment is covered only in outline in this book.

A series of diagnostic audiological tests is performed. Typically this includes pure-tone audiometry, speech audiometry, tympanometry, acoustic reflex tests, otoacoustic emissions or OAEs (in which the acoustic response from the outer hair cells is recorded) and auditory evoked electrical potentials (AEPs). The value of including AEPs measured from different points in the auditory pathway in the CI test battery is increasingly recognized (Cullington, 2002). The measures used in combination may help to distinguish between a site of lesion in which a CI may be beneficial (such as cases of absent inner hair cells but an intact auditory nerve) (Gibson, 2003; Rea and Gibson, 2003) and those in which a CI is contraindicated (e.g. as a result of a lesion or auditory neuropathy of the eighth nerve, auditory brain-stem dysfunction and/or central auditory pathology). Tests that have been reported as particularly useful in this regard are round window electrocochleography, which records the electrical responses triggered by the inner hair cells of the cochlea (Incerti et al., 2002), auditory brainstem response testing, which records the electrical activity of the eighth nerve, and brainstem and cortical evoked response testing. AEPs also help to verify auditory thresholds, particularly to identify cases of functional hearing loss or overlay (Spraggs et al., 1994) and rare cases of conversion deafness, i.e. unconscious manifestation of hearing loss (Balko et al., 2002), who occasionally present to implant programmes.

In some clinics, subjective responses to transtympanic electrical stimulation (a test known as the promontory stimulation test or PST) form part of the audiological assessment. The prognostic value of the latter test has recently been questioned (Chen et al., 2001). However, in cases where the patient demonstrates no measurable auditory thresholds in the ear considered for implantation, it may provide useful information for preoperative counselling and provide the patient with the reassuring psychophysical experience of hearing electrically stimulated sound. Kuo and Gibson (2002) reported that a group of implantees who perceived sound during promontory stimulation averaged a score of 81% on the Central Institute for the Deaf (CID) speech tests compared with 42% for the small group of patients who were unable to hear sound when electrical current was delivered to the round window. In some programmes, the important contribution of vestibular assessment to the decision to implant one ear or the other has been highlighted. Implanting the only ear with any labyrinthine function could result in bilateral vestibular loss and chronic ataxia (Chen et al., 2001; Gibson, 2003). This is particularly important in older CI recipients whose adaptation to changed vestibular input may be slower. In summary, suitable candidates will show an overall pattern of results consistent with a cochlear site of lesion at moderate sloping to profound levels or worse.

If the patient is able to detect speech using hearing aids, an assessment of aided speech recognition is performed in the 'best-aided' condition, i.e. with the optimal hearing aid fitting. Aided assessment is also essential for demonstrating changes in performance as a result of the cochlear implant. The postoperative assessment is described in more detail in Chapter 4.

Best-aided condition

The term 'best-aided condition' implies that the hearing aid fitting has been reviewed and optimized. The best-aided performance may be obtained from either an individual ear or a binaural fitting. This may include the fitting and trial of appropriately styled ear moulds as well as appropriate amplification and assistive listening devices (ALDs). In some cases several appointments may be required. An optimal fitting may require the patient to try an alternative hearing aid, binaural devices or a combination of hearing aids plus ALDs (e.g. a hearing aid coupled with an FM listening device or hand-held microphone). With the recent introduction of power digital hearing aids and a reduction in the audiometric criteria for implantation (i.e. patients with more residual hearing are being considered), the optimal fit may be a digital device. Recruitment (the abnormal growth in perception of loudness above threshold) may limit the usefulness or acceptability of analogue devices by some patients. In our experience, patients who were unable to tolerate an analogue device as a result of a severely reduced dynamic range, even with appropriate and adequate limiting, may be successfully fitted with power digital devices. This may be a result of the flexibility of these devices in tailoring the gain and output in specific frequency bands.

In addition, some patients may require a period of auditory training for the best-aided condition to be attained. Typically, such patients are those who have not recently worn hearing aids when presenting to the clinic, and borderline candidates undergoing trials of new amplification devices, whose aided measures may fall just outside the manufacturer's criterion. Patients who have been unaided for extended periods would require an extended period of acclimatization to optimize the fitting. The patient's local rehabilitationist can play an important role in ensuring that an adequate trial of revised hearing aids has taken place.

As stated earlier in the chapter, the goal of the programme is to find a solution to the patient's hearing problem. A programme that encourages the implant candidate to access all existing technology in the process of assessment means that the patient can confidently make a well-informed decision. Some clinics carry a stock of devices that can be loaned to the patients for the purposes of evaluation. The process of optimizing the hearing aid fitting provides other valuable information about the patient to the CI team. This includes insight into the following:

- How well the patient manages additional information and new auditory or tactile sensations.
- How much support the patient needs to cope with and learn to use new devices.
- The patient's levels of perseverance: is he or she looking for a quick fix or willing to try different solutions?
- The patient's ability to integrate the new information with lip-reading.

Aided speech recognition assessment

The aided speech recognition assessment establishes whether the patient meets the criteria for implantation in the best-aided condition. Criteria for cochlear implant candidacy are based on analysis of the postoperative speech recognition performance of large groups of patients using the proposed device. Increasingly, there is more general agreement between centres on suitability criteria. Clinics may be guided by CI manufacturers' guidelines, regulatory bodies such as the Food and Drug Administration in the USA (FDA), major cochlear implant centres and the quality standards documents of national organizations such as the British Cochlear Implant Group (BCIG), e.g. the current candidacy criteria for the Cochlear Ltd Contour device include the criterion that open-set scores for word (recognition) in sentences, audition alone, do not exceed 60% in the ear to be implanted (Cochlear Ltd, 2004).

Alternative criteria may be used when assessing candidates who fall outside a conventional candidacy point but have a poorer ear that could very well receive significant benefit from an implant. Winton et al. (2002) proposed criteria for open-set sentence scores of less than 70% in the best-aided condition and less than 40% in the ear to be implanted. In a retrospective study evaluating the appropriateness of these criteria for postlingually deafened adults who achieved some speech understanding preoperatively, it was found that all patients showed an improvement with the implant compared with the pre-implant speech perception score with the hearing aid in the implanted ear. Post-implant scores also surpassed the non-implanted ear-aided scores for all but 15% of patients. This highlights the need for a holistic approach that considers factors such as patient history, additional handicaps, lifestyle and maintaining the patient's livelihood. Timely provision of an implant in such borderline cases may allow a patient to continue to work – a far better prospect than re-employment or retraining down the track.

Aided speech perception testing is usually performed in a sound-treated room using standardized (audio or video recorded) materials. Although live voice presentation may be used, the results must be viewed with some caution as a result of possible presenter bias. The actual tests employed vary for prelingually and postlingually deafened adults, as well as from clinic to clinic, but the test conditions should be similar. Typically, the tests include aided, sound-field, warble-tone thresholds, and detection and discrimination of phonemes, words and words in the context of sentences (in quiet and in noise). Measures of the patient's word (in sentence) recognition with and without lip-reading may be employed to assess the contribution of the auditory signal to speech recognition with visual cues and the patient's ability to integrate these modes. Measures with each ear separately, as well as binaural measures, may provide information to assist the patient and CI team to select the most appropriate ear for implantation (see p. 25). The reader is referred to Dowell et al. (1990) for a discussion of assessment materials.

Which ear to implant?

Should candidacy be identified, it is important for the CI team to inform the patient of any findings that suggest that one ear may be more suitable for implantation than the other. Examples include findings related to the computed tomography (CT) scan, asymmetrical vestibular function or asymmetrical, individual ear aided, speech perception scores. In our experience, where speech perception is poor bilaterally (i.e. < 30% on open-set sentences), implanting the better ear can lead to better outcomes. Lack of hearing aid use in one ear for more than 20 years, with consistent hearing aid use in the other ear, may also influence choice of ear. Clinics differ in their preference to implant the better- or worse-hearing ear. However, a report by Chen et al. (2001) suggests that the outcome is not significantly affected by this choice 'provided that the historical background of the hearing loss in the two ears is not very different'. The patient's involvement in this decision is very important. Patients should be clearly informed that residual hearing in the implanted ear could be lost, because this may affect not only choice of ear but whether a patient decides to continue with implantation at that time. In addition, clarification about continued use of a hearing aid in the other ear may be a deciding factor for the patient. This is discussed further in Chapter 3.

With an increase worldwide in bilateral cochlear implantation, and reported advantages for speech understanding in noise (Muller et al., 2002) and horizontal sound localization (Verschuur and Lutman, 2003), future implant candidates and CI teams may also need to discuss whether to implant one or both ears.

Otolaryngology assessment

The aim of this chapter is not to discuss the medical aspects of cochlear implant assessment in detail, but to note its position in the total assessment procedure. (Tucci and Niparko (2000) provide a more detailed account for the interested reader.) In the otological assessment, the patient's fitness for surgery is assessed and the patient is examined for any medical contraindications to implantation or for any conditions that require treatment before implant surgery such as middle-ear pathology. High-resolution CT of the inner ear and temporal bone is arranged to provide information about cochlear patency (and, hence, the likelihood of complete insertion of the electrode), structural changes to the temporal bone, particularly inner-ear deformities, and to identify any aetiology that may predispose the patient to adventitious stimulation of the facial nerve. The last is not necessarily a contraindication to implantation but may affect patient counselling and postoperative device programming.

Rehabilitation assessment

This part of the assessment is concerned with assessing (1) the patient and support partner's level of knowledge and understanding of all of the information that has been presented to them up to this point, (2) the patient's wider communication needs, (3) the patient's communication skills, (4) the patient's psychological strengths and weaknesses, (5) the support network available and (6) the patient's and the partner's attitude to implantation. This information is likely to be gathered over a series of appointments. The team's professionals involved may include an audiologist, a rehabilitationist (such as a hearing therapist), a psychologist and/or a social worker. There are significant advantages to involving a local professional, e.g. the patient's local rehabilitationist can ensure that patients are fully aware of their local support network. Their local professional will be a key person in supporting the patient whether or not he or she becomes a CI user. Local professionals have usually known the patient for some time, possibly even years, and can provide the CI team with valuable insights into the patient's difficulties and alert the team to any areas of concern.

Communication assessment

The aim is to assess the patient's broader communication needs and abilities. The appointments in this stage involve an active process of two-way information sharing. Clinicians clearly have a responsibility to convey information to their patient. Equally important is the clinician's active listening role, i.e. paying attention to not only what the patient reports, but *how* it is reported. It is reasonable to expect the patient to have read the introductory information provided. The intimacy of the one-on-one sessions will reveal any misconceptions that patients may have about the likely outcome with a CI, their understanding of the technical information, their level of interest in the CI, and their communication abilities and style. Prompts that may be used at this stage include 'What do you hope to achieve with a CI?', 'In what ways do you think life/your lifestyle will be better with a CI?', 'What difference do you think the CI will make to your communication ability?' and 'Do you have a willing support partner who will assist you throughout the process?' In many cases the deafness may cause the patient's life to come to a 'standstill'. It can be revealing to ask both the patients and their partners to speculate how their life and relationship may change post-implant.

In addition, the patient's home, work and social situations are discussed and difficulties in communication in each of these situations assessed. The extent to which hearing-impaired individuals have withdrawn from communication and become isolated is identified. The patient's relationship and communication with family and friends is discussed to ascertain the role of the individual within the family. The extent to which the family understand the patient's needs and the level of support available should be ascertained. It is helpful to identify the patient's professional support network at this stage, to ensure that all professionals currently involved with the patient's health and welfare are supportive of the assessment for a CI.

The assessment should include the patient's awareness of, and need for, other communication devices such as environmental alerting aids, vibrating alarms for the alarm clock, vibrating pagers, loop systems, TTY, Teletext, fax machines, etc. This assessment will also evaluate the patient's use and awareness of communication and conversation strategies and tactics (see Chapter 7). The information obtained will help to structure the patient's postoperative communication training. Any other factors affecting communication, such as expressive language difficulties brought about by a stroke, should be identified. A referral to a speech and language therapist may be indicated in some cases (see Chapter 8).

Communication profiles and quality-of-life (QoL) self-assessment measures specific to hearing disability may provide information about the candidate's functional communication ability and form an important part of assessing the patient preoperatively. The Glasgow Benefit Inventory (GBI) (Robinson et al., 1996) measures quality of life, focusing on independence levels, personal and social relationships and adjustment to deafness. Hawthorne and Hogan (2002) reported on the use of a revised (shortened) version of the Glasgow Hearing Status Inventory. This 11-item instrument measures self-esteem, social handicap and hearing handicap. These measures provide a baseline of the patient's situation preoperatively and can be repeated post-implant to assess in which dimensions improvements have occurred.

The Communication Profile for the Hearing Impaired (CPHI) (Demorest and Erdman, 1987) is an assessment tool for communication skills, including communication strategies, communication effectiveness at home and work, and personal adjustment such as acceptance of loss and withdrawal. Binzer (2000) suggests that the CPHI is a valid tool for assessment of coping and adjustment to hearing impairment by CI users post-implant, but cautions that an explanation to the CI recipient about the intent of some questions is required.

Clinicians interested in measuring improvements in conversational performance pre- and post-therapy may consider using DYALOG (Erber, 1998). This computer software can be used to evaluate live or video-taped conversation and provide a measure of the time spent in communication breakdown, the number of repair events and the average time per event.

Psychological assessment

A psychologist (or psychotherapist) contributes a wider perspective to the CI team by looking at how patients interact with the world around them. In some clinics, every patient undergoes a comprehensive psychological assessment both before and after implantation so that a full picture of the CI candidate is built up and the long-term impact of implantation can be assessed (Aplin, 1993). Where resources are more restricted, the psychologist may be required to see patients only where there are concerns (such as a depressive illness) or where a questionnaire indicates significant psychological needs. For a newly established programme, however, we would recommend that all patients undergo a psychological evaluation initially, until the CI team gains more experience.

It should be stressed that identifying a problem or need during the psychological assessment does not necessarily exclude a patient from being implanted. Rather the aim is to provide the team with information that will assist in the *management* of the patient and family during this period of change. The actual assessment tools vary from clinic to clinic. These may include measures of specific cognitive abilities such as vigilance (Knutson et al., 1991), general intelligence measures, personality profiles and counselling profiles. For an outline of assessment techniques the reader is referred to Aplin (1993). With tools that depend heavily on verbal administration (e.g. the relevant verbal subtests of the Wechsler Adult Intelligence Scale or WAIS-III – Wechlser, 1997), it can be helpful to present the material in written format.

In most cases, the verbal and non-verbal intellectual abilities of patients are assessed. This allows insight into problem-solving ability, and ability to follow instructions, attend to detail, and manage different learning and, possibly, frustrating situations, plus the patient's response to challenging situations. These areas are important, because one of the roles of psychological assessment is to identify those patients who may not cope with the postoperative procedures involved (Clark et al., 1977). The intellectual assessment also provides information about a candidate's other cognitive strengths and weakness, so that they may either be capitalized on (e.g. long attention span), or worked around (e.g. reduced short-term memory) in the rehabilitation period. An assessment of the candidate's vocabulary level is important so that the literacy level of test materials, consent forms and auditory training material, for example, is appropriate.

The psychologist's input provides information about the patient's interests, lifestyle, interpersonal relationships and family support. Other aspects that may be explored include personality characteristics and ability to adapt to change. Changes or psychological trauma, such as adjustment to deafness, affecting both the individual and relationships, can be discussed. It is useful to identify if the patient has had or is currently experiencing any symptoms of emotional disorder such as depression because this may require management before or after implantation.

The patient's motivation for seeking implantation and the changes that he or she hopes the implant will bring about will be discussed. This is extremely important because, if the desired changes are unrealistic, use of the implant is unlikely to be reinforced (McKenna, 1991). The psychologist may form an opinion as to how easily the patient is likely to adjust to the implant and maintain it. Factors that may impede learning or adjustment post-implant can be made known to the rehabilitation team so that the patient's expectations can be adjusted accordingly. With older patients, the psychologist may look for evidence of deterioration of cognitive function. The psychologist can explore concerns that other members of the team have raised during assessment. Any psychologist new to the area of implantation should be provided with a clear remit of the areas that the team requires them to explore. The following prompts for a structured interview may be helpful:

- How does the patient feel about his or her deafness?
- How has the patient coped with being a deafened adult? What impact has deafness had on the individual and his or her family? What adjustments have had to be made?
- Will having a CI fulfil his or her expectations for hearing, as well as for social and emotional functioning and employment needs?
- Has the patient experienced any depressive or anxiety symptoms that are being masked by the level of deafness?
- What is the patient's learning style? What adjustments to the rehabilitation programme may be required?
- Does he or she have any additional needs that the team should be alerted to, such as limitations in literacy? Does the patient have poor memory or any cognitive problems?
- Does the patient have any hidden agendas: is he or she honest and straightforward?
- How does he or she cope with disappointment or setbacks?
- What is his or her level of motivation? What evidence can the patient provide of long-term commitment to other projects?
- Is there anything in the medical history (e.g. previous or current mental health issues) that might make it difficult to manage the long-term commitment, or that might cause the patient to reject the CI or hinder him or her from working with the team?
- What are the patient's priorities with respect to goal setting? Are these consistent with the CI team's assessment of likely outcomes?

- Is the relationship with his or her partner under stress? Would relationship counselling be of assistance?

Managing expectations

A little knowledge can be a dangerous thing!

In our experience, adult cochlear implant candidates arrive at the implant centre with considerably more knowledge about cochlear implants than they did 5 years ago. Many patients have already met someone who has a CI. Patients may have read articles about, or written by, CI users in newspapers, magazines and on TV. There are a growing number of books describing personal experiences with a CI. Information technology has vastly facilitated the layperson's access to technical CI information. All CI manufacturers have internet sites with 'most frequently asked questions'. In addition there are email chat sites and CI forums where users, non-users and prospective candidates can discuss the relative merits of different implant systems.

Although implant candidates may be better informed, and possibly more positive and motivated, the downside of this is that patients are more likely to have preconceived and heightened expectations of the outcomes of implantation, particularly if they have met or read about a 'star' CI user. Many patients believe that if they work hard enough with the CI they will achieve their goals or match the abilities of CI users whom they have met.

The goals of expectation counselling are twofold: first, to identify the patient's and support person's current expectations and knowledge and, second, to modify those expectations through the provision of a more realistic and balanced picture. This is a process rather than a one-off event. The process begins with the patient's introductory information session, is supported by the provision of written information and continues through discussions with the psychologist, rehabilitationist and other CI recipients. During this process, the patient's understanding of the information and willingness to accept it is reviewed and refined by the team. Appropriate expectations are those that are *likely* to be achieved given the individual's presenting history. As stated above, if the implant provides the changes that the patient expects, use of the implant will be reinforced.

Identification of current knowledge can be achieved through open-ended questions such as the following:

- What do you hope to achieve from the cochlear implant?
- How long do you think it will take to achieve this?
- What are your ideas about how speech might sound through the implant?
- How useful do you expect the implant to be for understanding conversation?

- How well do you expect to follow television programmes?
- Do you think it is likely that you will be able to have telephone conversations using the implant?
- How important will lip-reading and other tactics be after receiving an implant?
- How do you expect music to sound through a cochlear implant?

The advantages of including the support person in the counselling process have already been discussed. If the support person understands that the sound quality from the implant is not optimal at switch-on, this provides an opportunity to discuss the on-going need for good communication skills to supplement the implant in the early stages, and to discourage the family from 'testing' the CI user without visual cues – an activity likely to lead to disappointment all round. Detailed suggestions for family counselling at the switch-on period are made in Chapter 3.

The next two sections address the areas that may concern a clinician beginning in this field. First, specific examples of what a CI recipient may reasonably expect from an implant are described. Second, different approaches are suggested to communicate this information.

What to expect from a cochlear implant

The clinician's role is to provide a balanced picture that is realistic, yet positive. It can be useful to relate each of the points below back to the candidate's current position and how this might be improved with an implant. The following areas of discussion are pivotal to avoiding disappointment later.

Implications of implanting the best/worse ear

It can save considerable counselling (and patient anxiety) if any medical contraindications to implanting either ear are known at this point so that only the options *available* can be fully explored. Examples include middle-ear disease, inner-ear disease or deformity and uncertainty about eighth nerve integrity. In cases where the better functioning ear has been recommended from a medical perspective, a patient's reluctance to implant this ear is understandable – it is their lifeline for communication with the world. Although the risks of surgical complications are minimal, it is a real concern to some candidates who will welcome frank discussion. Anxiety about communicating *without* the better ear for up to 4 weeks after surgery may affect the patient's decision to implant it. The clinician can emphasize the relatively short duration of this period in the whole programme and suggest coping strategies. The patient should be aware of individual ear factors relating to his or her clinical history (amount of residual hearing, consistent use of hearing aids, PST results) that may impact on the range of outcomes, as discussed above. Many clinics discourage use of amplification in the non-implanted ear initially after switch-on, because adaptation to the implant signal may be facilitated through focus on listening through the CI alone (see Chapter 3 for further discussion). This is an issue here because some flexibility may help a patient to decide which ear to proceed with. Although the team may make a recommendation, at the end of the day it is the patient who must weigh up the pros and cons, and ultimately live with the decision.

Initial sound quality

The patient should be aware that the quality of the sound though the CI after switch-on can be poor, because this awareness may reduce the initial disappointment. However, the clinician should emphasize that the sound quality improves over time, often quite markedly over the first few days and weeks. The contributions that regular speech processor programming and listening practice can make to accelerate this process can be discussed.

Understanding speech in quiet

Many postlingually deafened adults are now achieving impressive accuracy on speech recognition tasks without visual cues. One-on-one conversation *in quiet* is described as 'almost effortless' by many of our CI recipients and their spouses. However, counselling on the range of possible outcomes should take into consideration the candidates' preoperative speech understanding. Dowell et al. (2002) reported that postlingually deafened adults who demonstrated consistent hearing aid use and obtained some speech-perception benefit (10% or more) before implantation scored significantly higher on sentences in quiet (75% scored above 68%) and had better outcomes than recipients who demonstrated no preoperative speech-perception benefit.

The contribution of speech reading

In our experience congenitally deafened adults show a considerable range in outcomes for understanding speech without visual cues, from those with no open-set recognition to some who recognize more than half of the words in sentences without lip-reading. However, most report reduced *dependence* on visual cues with implant use over time, once they have learned to use the new auditory cues. CI users frequently report being more relaxed during communication and less tired at the end of the day, compared with their preoperative status, a change that many CI recipients attribute to the reduced effort required for lip-reading. However, the need to continue to supplement the implant sound with visual cues, especially when speaker characteristics or acoustics are not ideal, should be emphasized. It is important to ensure that the support person understands that the need for visual cues will not disappear.

Hearing in background noise or in group situations

Noise will continue to present some listening difficulties for CI recipients. However, it should be emphasized that many CI users report an improvement in these situations compared with the hearing aid, and further improvement over time. This may be the result of experience (resulting in increased tolerance of noise), optimization of the speech processor program and parameters, structured auditory training in noise and the CI recipient's developing ability to optimize the processor settings and/or use appropriate assistive devices.

Environmental sounds

The advantages of being able to *detect* environmental sounds, such as an item dropped on the floor or a car approaching, should be balanced with an understanding that learning to *recognize* the sounds occurs with experience and time and *localization* of sounds is not always possible. A wide range of environmental sounds should be identifiable to a CI user within the first few months of CI use. Some sounds are more easily distinguishable than others, e.g. the phone ringing is relatively easy because of its pattern code and is often identified within the first few days. Compare this with bird song, which, because it is higher pitched and irregular in pattern, may take longer to be recognized. New CI users can be overwhelmed by the amount of sound around them soon after switch-on. One patient recalled this time as one of 'sensory overload' with many sounds being heard, but with difficulty distinguishing between foreground and background sounds. Some sounds may continue to be irritating for some time until an increased level of tolerance is developed. Important positive aspects are increased independence through recognition of alerting sounds, feeling more 'in touch with the world' and the fact that many CI recipients report hearing *soft* environmental sounds for the first time in many years.

Voice monitoring

Cochlear implant users will hear their own voice as soon as the implant is switched on, but may not recognize it at first, particularly those with long duration of profound or total deafness. Many CI recipients do not like the sound of their own voice initially and comment on the loudness of their own voice compared with other speakers' voices. Improved voice level monitoring follows naturally within a few hours or days for most CI recipients. Articulation improves for some patients (see Chapter 8 for more detail on changes in the speech of CI recipients post-implant).

Following television programmes

It is difficult to predict how well clients will follow speech on TV because it is affected by the type of programmes watched (programmes with greater amounts of face to camera such as news programmes are easier than dramas with foreign accents, background music and lighting effects). CI candidates should be prepared for understanding of TV speech to take longer than 'live voice' speech. Older implant recipients appear to have greater difficulty following fast and degraded (e.g. accented) speech, perhaps caused by diminishing central auditory processing and/or cognitive skills. It is therefore important to prepare older implant candidates, for the possibility that they may continue to be reliant on Teletext and/or assistive devices (e.g. those that provide direct input from the TV to the speech processor).

Telephone use

The ability to use the telephone is highly dependent on the ability to hear speech without relying on visual cues. Providing the patient with accurate counselling on this issue can be difficult because some patients, who present with good prognostic indicators, can demonstrate poor open-set speech recognition immediately after switch-on. Generally speaking, the longer the duration of profound loss and period of auditory deprivation, the less chance there is that the patient will discriminate well over the phone. This is discussed in more detail in Chapter 10. Phone use is often a very emotive issue; many patients strongly desire the independence of being able to make and receive their own phone calls, and the inexperienced clinician may feel pressured into making promises that cannot be realized. Caution is recommended, perhaps emphasizing the range of outcomes, and the possibility of circumventing some of the auditory limitations through skilled use of communication strategies such as limited-choice questions. For all patients, the ability to use the phone will depend on the patient's ability to supplement his or her speech recognition abilities (auditory alone), together with clarification and conversational management strategies when he or she cannot understand the speaker (see Chapters 7 and 10).

Most CI recipients report some limitations to phone use, e.g. a patient who can converse with family and friends may still have difficulty understanding an unfamiliar speaker on the telephone. However, in our experience, developments in speech processors, processing strategies and telephone-specific ALDs (see Chapter 10) are making telephone conversation through an implant a possibility for increasing numbers of CI recipients.

It is essential to explore any hidden agendas with respect to phone use. A patient's wish to be able to make emergency calls (where the patient can get largely by *giving* information) and the occasional social call to a family member may be realistic. However, a patient whose aim is to regain the use of the phone for work to expand career prospects will need careful expectation counselling.

Music

It is difficult to counsel objectively in the area of potential benefits of implantation to the enjoyment of music. Many CI recipients do regain their enjoyment of music through the implant, although the *degree* of enjoyment is wide-ranging. Individual patients have reported resuming playing the piano, enjoying orchestral concerts and participating in sung church services. Some CI recipients strongly dislike the sound of music through the implant, however. Open-set melody recognition continues to be very difficult for most CI recipients, even when rhythm cues are available (Gfeller et al., 2002).

A great deal depends on the *importance* of music to the individual and this should be fully explored at this time. Those wishing to be able to hear music as a comforting background sound are less likely to be disappointed than a patient who has a discerning appreciation of classical music, or whose profession is music based, and those who play an instrument. Most commonly, patients report that music quality is somewhat limited but enjoy the fact that they can hear it clearly enough to *participate* again in social events such as church services, singing 'Happy Birthday' with their children, Christmas carols, etc.

Most patients report that the quality of music improves over time, e.g. the rhythm of the music may be discerned quite soon after switch-on, but hearing the melody or the words to a song may take several months. Anecdotal reports suggest that those who regularly make time to listen to music through the implant are rewarded for their efforts. In some cases, changes to the programming of the device can improve the perception of music. However, it should be emphasized that the implant was designed first and foremost to improve verbal communication. Refinements to the sound processing software and processing algorithms aimed specifically at music are likely to bring increased benefit in listening to music in future years. However, these benefits may not be available retrospectively to patients with earlier implant/speech processor models.

Education and employment

Increasingly, the benefits of implantation extend to the workplace. In a qualitative study (Hogan et al., 2002), CI recipients reported more confidence, and greater job satisfaction and independence in the workplace post-implant. Specific benefits reported by CI recipients at our centres include being able to follow instructions without reliance on others, increased awareness of alerting/warning sounds (feedback from computers, when a fax arrives or that a machine has stopped) and feelings of increased inclusion at break times. There are increasing numbers of CI recipients performing well in complex and noisy working environments, coping with meetings and using the telephone in the workplace, but these are currently in the minority.

The clinician should be cautious, however, with regard to the client hoping for significant career changes or promotion, to gain further training or avoid retrenchment. It is important to establish the importance of such goals and the underlying motive (see Chapter 9). Although there are individual cases of CI recipients securing better-paid employment or a more satisfying position, there are no certainties. In fact, it has been reported that CI users required considerable support to enable them to get back into employment or to optimize their employment opportunities (Hogan et al., 1999; Hogan, 2001).

Tinnitus

Many patients with tinnitus are concerned about possible changes to tinnitus perception post-implant. For many adults, the tinnitus is ameliorated by having a CI in either the same or the other ear (Hazell et al., 1989; Gibson, 1992; Summerfield and Marshall, 1995). It is important to clarify the difference between a patient's tinnitus being ameliorated (i.e. a masking effect where the tinnitus is less audible in the presence of the sound from the implant) and being cured or resolved by implantation. When the tinnitus is masked by sound from the implant, the patient may learn to pay less attention to it over time. In patients who express concerns about postoperative tinnitus, it may be wise to prepare them for the possibility of the tinnitus increasing immediately postoperatively and for a few days after switch-on. In rare cases the tinnitus may be exacerbated on a long-term basis.

Cochlear implants improve only hearing status

Any suggestions that the CI will improve personality traits or communication disorders must be challenged, because when these desired changes do not occur the implant is likely to be regarded as a failure, regardless of any improvements in communication. Any concerns in this area should be referred to the appropriate professional for further assessment.

Time factors

The patient should have a clear understanding of the timeframe involved. The implant is not a 'quick fix'. Establishing stable current levels to provide an audible but comfortable level of stimulation is affected by both physiological changes in the newly implanted cochlear and practice effects with the mapping procedures. This may take several weeks. The patient should understand that the information provided by the implant is sometimes incomplete and that a variety of skills will need to be learned to supplement the incomplete message (see Chapters 5, 6 and 7). Not all implant candidates are initially aware that the implant is a life-long commitment, requiring mapping at least once a year for the client's lifetime.

Counselling pre- and perilingually deafened adults

When counselling these groups, a broader definition of a successful outcome that does not focus on speech perception, but rather emphasizes other quality-of-life attributes, has been found to be helpful. Young congenitally deafened adults may explore the implant option when on the threshold of independence, separating from parents, entering the workforce or further education, desiring to travel or widening their social contacts. The benefits reported by this group have provided useful discussion points for counselling and include increased environmental awareness, especially for soft or high-frequency sounds, 'feeling safer', improved voice monitoring, increased use of voice, enhanced cues for appropriate social interaction (e.g. awareness of emotional content and/or speaker intent), assistance with lip-reading, increased self-confidence, increased independence, reduced sense of isolation and greater ease of learning new vocabulary (Rushbrooke and Pedley, 2002). Although entrenched patterns of speech production would be unlikely to change as a result of a CI, improved articulation after intense speech and language therapy has occurred in a small number of cases. In our experience, the support and appropriate expectations of the family are pivotal to success.

Approaches to discussing expectations

Given that patients are grappling with technical information, practical choices, medical issues, financial considerations, potential outcomes and their own severely impaired communication, it is not surprising that expectations need to be discussed more than once for the patients to understand fully the likely outcomes with a CI device and the possible limitations for use. Providing this information in several different ways, from different members of the team, increases the likelihood that the relevant information has been understood. There are many ways to provide opportunities for patients to develop appropriate expectations and these are discussed in more detail below. The use of at least two of these approaches is recommended with each patient. These could include:

- meeting an experienced CI recipient and his or her support person
- use of questionnaires
- family counselling
- video recordings.

Meeting a CI recipient and support person

There are many advantages to candidates from meeting CI users, as long as the meeting is well managed. If efforts are made to match the CI user where possible to the adult patient with a similar onset and duration of profound deafness, the meeting can be very beneficial to the CI recipient (and the family). For some individuals it is important to take gender, lifestyle and particularly age of the CI user into consideration for the meeting to be relevant. It is important that the clinician explains to the CI candidate exactly where similarities and differences in performance with the CI user might be anticipated.

Candidates can receive a first-hand account of everyday experiences from the CI user and learn whether the CI recipient considered the process worthwhile. Discussing the outcome of a CI first hand provides a highly credible description of issues of high concern such as: what the sound is really like through a CI, how long it took to adjust and the circumstances under which the CI recipient can and cannot hear. Meeting an implant recipient can convey the improvement that many CI recipients gain in everyday conversation better than any written testimony; the ease with which the CI recipient participates is often in stark contrast to the candidate's struggle to follow the discussion. Many candidates have a particular fear or concern, and sometimes this surfaces for the first time in this interview (e.g. 'How much did the scar hurt afterwards?', 'How did you get by without any hearing aid while you were awaiting switch-on?'). Patients often appear to be more reassured by a CI recipient than by the professionals on the team. They may find comfort in knowing that the CI recipient had similar concerns or fears before his or her own surgery. Spouses, in particular, take great comfort from sharing the frustrations and difficulties of communication before implantation and hearing first hand how many of these burdens were reduced post-implant.

The main disadvantage is that unrealistic expectations may be set up because either the candidate and user were not well matched for likely outcome (the use of 'excellent performers' is discouraged for this reason), or the candidate fails to appreciate the time needed to arrive at this level of communication ability or other outcome. In the worse case, this can lead to discouragement and poor use post-implant.

Sensitive, perceptive and articulate CI recipients are particularly good in this role. It has been suggested that severely hearing-impaired people communicate more openly and frankly with others with a significant hearing loss than with a clinician who has not personally experienced deafness. Providing training and support for CI users who are willing to support the clinic in this way is one way to enhance the process (Gailey, 2000). Feedback from the meeting is incorporated into the team's assessment of the patient and the team can plan to meet any concerns that still need to be addressed. If this meeting takes place without a member of the CI team, a volunteer CI recipient should have clear guidelines about the extent of the role. The clinic should have clear guidelines on the exchange of personal details.

Facilitating a meeting with an experienced CI user

The seating and lighting arrangements for the room are similar to those described for the information session. Seating around a small coffee table is ideal, because it helps to provide a more intimate setting for discussion of personal matters while at the same time providing a barrier so that people do not feel quite so 'exposed'.

As communication with strangers presents an additional challenge, the clinician can facilitate by offering to rephrase comments, write down key words or take notes during the session for reading later. Profoundly deaf candidates, who expend so much energy just following the communication, really appreciate this facilitation, because they are then better able to consider the replies.

Sufficient time should be allowed for all parties to establish a rapport and for the inevitable breakdowns in communication. A minimum of half an hour is recommended. The candidate and family should be advised of the time available and should be encouraged to prepare their questions in advance.

After introductions, the easiest way to begin is to invite the candidate to ask questions. This allows the candidate to introduce the topics for discussion, making comprehension of replies easier. The clinician may choose to stay throughout the meeting to ensure that the candidate gets the opportunity to ask questions. On the other hand, the clinician may decide to leave the room periodically to allow discussion of more private matters or issues that the candidate may feel are too 'basic' to be raised in front of a professional. A candidate with considerable communication difficulties should be supported by a clinician throughout, because otherwise the burden of interpretation falls on the support person who may then not have the opportunity to ask his or her own questions.

At the close of the session, the clinician should ensure that all of the candidate's questions have been asked. In our experience, this process is very satisfying for the experienced CI recipients and their support people because their own communication ability and confidence with the implant are a testimony to their progress. Some CI recipients will offer ongoing support to the candidate and the family.

Use of questionnaires to assess and modify expectations and assess candidacy

Clinicians may use a questionnaire to check the understanding and expectations of implant candidates and their support partners at the end of the assessment and counselling process. CI manufacturers provide some tools to assist with assessing expectation. In our experience, use of the Code–Muller protocol (CMP) has been particularly helpful for working with clients. The application of the CMP is detailed in Hogan (2001). Ideally, the questionnaire will have separate versions for the candidate and support person. If the questionnaire has not been posted to the candidate's home, time should be allowed for completion of the forms at the clinic in a quiet area. The clinician and family then discuss the answers together, paying particular attention to any replies that indicate unrealistic expectations and any discrepancies between the expectations of the patient and support person.

Alternatively, the questions may be presented by the clinician 'interview style' with the responses recorded verbatim. This encourages the clinician to listen rather than to deliver monologues. The clinician may record any counselling given on each item and the final 'agreed or accepted' expectation. This may be provided later to the patient in written format as a record of the discussion. The recording of patient and family expectations is important for several reasons:

- It provides a record of the expectations for comparison with post-implant performance. This is useful if the patient develops unrealistic expectations after implantation and for the clinic to monitor the accuracy of the counselling provided.
- It provides a tool for moving towards 'closure' (see Chapter 9), when the patient can read that the agreed goals have been met.
- It provides documentation when the expectations need to be modified as a result of particular issues highlighted by the psychologist or other team members.
- Formally recording the agreed expectations can bring to light any discrepancies between what the clinician said and what the patient perceived.

Family counselling

A family counselling session, at either the clinic or the family home, is another way to clarify and confirm the expectations of the partner, support person and family. A checklist (see Appendices 2 and 3) is useful at this stage to ensure that all the items described above are covered. This checklist can also be used to obtain signed consent from the patient and support partner (see page 47).

Video recordings

Some clinics use an edited subtitled video recording of different consenting patients in the initial post-implant stages, describing the sound through the implant and how the sound changed over the ensuing weeks and months. This approach provides a range of outcomes and experiences to be communicated. The video may be used to show the tasks involved in the mapping procedure. When such videos are available to take home, the patient's family and support network can benefit.

Managing unrealistic expectations

If a patient continues to harbour expectations that the CI team consider unrealistic, in that they are unlikely to be achieved by that individual, the team should not proceed further with the assessment until these issues have been addressed. The team has several options:

- 'Straight talking' with the patient and support partner: it may be necessary for another member of the team to become involved, e.g. the team coordinator or patient's implant surgeon. Their role is to review

with the patient the concerns held by the team and to state reasons for
the expected outcome with a CI.

- Offer the chance for the patient to meet a matched CI user: this may help
  to get the message across especially if the CI user is asked to comment on
  the limitations of the device.
- Arrange a meeting with a psychologist: there may be complex issues for
  the patient that a psychologist might be able to explore further.
- Defer the decision to implant: this is not necessarily the best option, but
  does allow a 'cooling-off period' for patients to reassess their situation. It
  also makes a clear statement that the CI team are not prepared to proceed
  further until this issue has been resolved.

Practical considerations

This section describes some of the practical issues that are addressed
through information counselling during the pre-implant period.

Choice of manufacturer's CI system

Clinics are increasingly offering patients a choice of CI systems from
different manufacturers. The relative merits of each device should be
discussed with the patient. Increasingly, when patients are making this
decision, they ask for information about options to update the external
components, internal device survival rates and comparative outcomes. The
availability of CI recipient chat sites and manufacturer's sites on the
worldwide web increases the likelihood that patients will consider more
than one device. If a patient has a strong preference for a particular implant
system, the clinician should check that the reasoning is sound.

Choice of style of device

This choice is concerned with the pros and cons of the ear-level and body-
worn speech processors for each patient. Generally, the cosmetic advantages
of an ear-level speech processor are important to adults, but it should not be
assumed that all adults would prefer this style of speech processor. The
wearing options, ergonomics and dexterity issues for each speech processor
should be explored using a demonstration device and considered in relation
to the patient's lifestyle. Information about access to customized speech-
processing strategies, number of listening programmes, special features such
as noise reduction and in-built telecoil, battery consumption and other
running costs should be presented so that the patient can make an informed
choice. More detailed information on practical issues of wearing the external
equipment can be found in Chapter 11.

Financial costs

The actual costs vary from country to country and are different between devices. They will depend on whether the patient covers all costs, and is treated under the public health system, and whether health authorities or medical insurers reimburse any expenses. The patient should be aware of any costs to themselves during the assessment and surgical period, the life-long costs of post-implant maintenance (including insurance, out-of-warranty repairs, batteries and spare parts) and local funding arrangements for upgrading the processor. For patients remote from the clinic, the cost of travel to the centre and accommodation need to be considered, together with local arrangements for reimbursement of such expenses, where applicable.

Limitations of using the device

It is essential to advise patients in writing of any restrictions on wearing the equipment, particularly those that would invalidate the manufacturer's warranty. This should include medical treatments such as magnetic resonance imaging and diathermy which may damage the internal device. The implant surgeon will advise that physical contact sports should be avoided as a blow to the head in the area of the implant may damage the internal device. Some implant surgeons also advise against scuba diving. The need to carry a registration card for identification as a CI user in the case of an accident may be mentioned at this point. Restrictions during air travel, such as the need to turn off the device when proceeding through airport security areas and during take-off and landing should be made clear. These are well documented (e.g. BCIG Safety Guidelines, 2003). The need to remove the external device before bathing and swimming, and the need for prompt and appropriate action should the external equipment get wet, should be outlined.

Surgery and hospital stay

The implant surgeon typically provides this information, but the team clinicians may be asked to clarify or confirm some points. Any concerns about these issues should be referred back to the surgeon. The patient is advised about the duration of surgery, which varies between clinics and surgeons. It may be helpful to advise the support partner that the patient will be away from the ward for a longer time than this because of recovery time after the surgery. Patients should be informed if shaving of hair will be necessary (this is usually a concern for female patients), the site and length of the operation scar and any postoperative discomfort (e.g. from the use of a pressure bandage). In some surgical approaches, patients may notice numbness over the implanted side of their head once the pressure bandage has been removed, which may persist for some months. However, feeling returns gradually to the pinna and numbness is mostly resolved by 4 weeks after surgery, around the time of switch-on. The usual length of hospital stay should be given together with typical recommendations for recovery time at home before returning to work.

Patients who wear spectacles can be advised to adjust a pair of spectacles by removing the spectacle arm on the implant side. This allows the patient to wear spectacles with the head bandage – an important consideration to those dependent on lip-reading. Once the postoperative swelling has reduced, the patient may be aware of a slightly raised area under the skin on the implanted side – the site of internal stimulus receiver package. Patients may require reassurance that it is perfectly normal to be able to feel the outline of the stimulus receiver plate through the skin. Patients are often keen to know how soon they can wash their hair after surgery. This should be checked with the surgeon or nursing staff before leaving hospital. In addition, the patient should be given clear information about whom to contact if they have any concerns after they have left the hospital. It can be to everyone's advantage if training in communication with severely deaf patients is offered to the ward staff and a sign indicating the patient's communication needs is provided by the bed.

Operation risks

The implant surgeon will explain the details of the surgery and the risks involved. Issues discussed may include anaesthesia, risk of facial nerve palsy, infection, haematoma, postoperative tinnitus, vertigo and changes to the sensation of taste.

Postoperative device programming and programming schedules

Patients should be given a broad outline of what is required of them during the programming of the device, how long this process normally takes and frequency of mapping appointments. Some programmes ask the patient to sign a copy of the agreed schedule of appointments. The consequences of non-attendance should be stated to the patient in terms that they can understand, such as 'the equipment requires regular fine-tuning to provide the best clarity and comfort, particularly in the early stages'. As discussed above, some patients find a video recording of a switch-on session helpful. Many of our patients have found it informative to sit in on part of a mapping session for an experienced patient. Considerations and practical suggestions for preparing the patient for switch-on are described in Chapter 3.

Research projects

Where the clinic has research commitments, particularly where the clinic's database of CI patients may be used retrospectively, the patient should be informed about the information collected and future plans to use these data. In some clinics, a consent form is used before switch-on. Where a patient is to be involved in a research study from the outset, it is important that the patient understands that withdrawal from any study would not compromise their ongoing care and support.

Bringing it all together

At the end of the assessment process, information has been gathered about the patient's medical, surgical, audiological and psychological suitability for implantation, together with an impression of the patient's and the family's expectations of the device, and their commitment to the implant programme.

This information must now be brought together to form a picture of the patient's overall suitability for implantation and likely benefits. This overall impression is used to provide the patient and family with an overview of the likely outcomes and any factors that may affect the post-implant rehabilitation.

There are a number of ways that this can be achieved. In some programmes, each team member provides a report and the implant surgeon conveys the information from all team members. In other programmes, the team members meet with the family in a 'round table' discussion. In a third model, the team members meet first without the family to present and discuss their findings and form a professional opinion of suitability and issues that may affect progress. This information is then shared with the candidate and family in a meeting that includes only the professionals who will be directly involved with the patient's post-implant care. Where the CI team is large, this last model has the benefit of drawing on the collective experience of many experienced professionals, including the patient in the decision-making process, but without the family being daunted or even intimidated by meeting a large group of people.

The final meeting with the implant candidate aims to convey the findings and opinion of each assessor, make a final decision about which ear is to be implanted and convey the team's opinion of the expected outcomes. Any factors identified as possibly affecting post-implant progress will be explained, and possible ways of reducing the impact may be outlined. The candidate and family have the opportunity to clarify any remaining concerns.

The family decides who attends this meeting. In addition to the key people from the family and the team, they may invite selected friends, relatives or neighbours who will be involved in rehabilitation, the patient's local professionals who will be involved in postoperative rehabilitation, work colleagues and even a member of a local support group. In many clinics, the family has a 'cooling-off' period after this meeting, during which they weigh up the information provided and reach a decision on the preferred course of management. Here are some examples:

> Alex was a congenitally profoundly hearing-impaired young adult presenting for implantation at the age of 24. His main motivation was the desire to live independently. He believed that being able to hear more environmental sounds and to communicate more easily with non-signing adults would help him to achieve this. The team indicated to Alex and his family that he was likely to gain assistance with lip-reading from the implant, increased awareness of environmental sounds and improved speech monitoring, but *not* increased speech intelligibility or understanding of speech without visual cues. The psychologist highlighted Alex's reduced social circle stemming from the family's recent move (and consequently the reduced opportunities for conversation practice) as a factor that may impact on initial progress. The team discussed avenues to provide increased social contact post-implant.
>
> Hannah was an elderly CI recipient whose profound hearing loss was relatively recent. Her main motivations for seeking implantation were to be able to participate more in family activities and to communicate with her grandchildren. Hannah and her family were counselled that there were no medical contraindications to surgery, and that both Hannah and family were likely to gain significantly from increased ease of communication, possibly without lip-reading, but that speed of progress may be affected by the decreased memory function noted in the assessment. The psychologist suggested reassessment of this factor post-implant. The rehabilitationist modified the post-implant rehabilitation to reduce the impact of this cognitive factor.
>
> Greg was a progressively deafened, binaurally aided, professional adult with a hearing loss that had recently reached profound levels. Greg was finding it increasingly difficult to cope in his office job and his main motivation for seeking implantation was to retain his livelihood and reduce the impact of the hearing loss on his marriage. Greg and his wife were counselled that the outcome for speech recognition was favourable, that understanding some speech on the telephone was likely but could not be guaranteed, and that return to work in an office position was not an unreasonable expectation. Greg's employer attended the final meeting and a staged return to work was agreed on to allow Greg time to become accustomed to the new sound sensations. An in-service training session for the work place was offered (see Chapters 6 and 9) to provide information to work colleagues and to explore possible modifications to Greg's work environment. The psychologist recommended a post-implant follow-up to explore relationship issues.
>
> Gloria was an adult perilingually deafened through meningitis who was an excellent speech reader but had not consistently worn hearing aids as a result of the limited benefit. Gloria hoped that a cochlear implant would improve her 'deaf speech' (which her mother had never come to terms with), help her to 'disguise' the deafness in public and allow her to talk with her family long distance on the

telephone. Despite expectation counselling from all team members, Gloria's expectations remained unrealistic. The team recommended deferring the decision to implant, further appointments with the psychologist to explore issues of identity and self-esteem were offered, and Gloria attended additional rehabilitation sessions to explore other communication technologies.

The use of signed consent

If the patient decides to proceed to implantation, the team may ask for consent forms to be signed. These may include permission to use data for research, the expected programme of appointments and a list of expectations personally tailored to address the likely outcome and any specific issues raised by the candidate. The use of signed consent is helpful in several ways:

- The use of a checklist ensures delivery of a quality standard of information for all patients in the programme.
- It makes a clear statement that the programme expects the patient and the support person to make a commitment to the programme to attend all appointments and to undertake the homework tasks if they wish to achieve maximum benefit from the CI.
- It provides a written record of issues concerning outcomes. This reduces the possibility of misunderstandings caused by the hearing loss and provides a reference later, should the patient's expectations become unrealistic.

Arrangements are then made to schedule surgery and switch-on.

Conclusion

This chapter has covered many issues in the assessment of potential cochlear implant candidates. A holistic approach involving a team of professionals has been emphasized. The advantages of involving a support person have been discussed. This approach emphasizes the needs and concerns of the patient and the benefits of ensuring that the patient fully participates in the decision process.

References

Aplin DY (1993) Psychological evaluation of adults in a cochlear implant program. American Annals of the Deaf 138: 415–19

Balko KA, Fordyce D, Blankenship K, Littman T, Backous D (2002) Conversion deafness in a cochlear implant patient. Poster presented at the 7th International Cochlear Implant Conference, Manchester UK, 4–6 September 2002

BCIG Safety Guidelines (2003) Recommended Guidelines on Safety for Cochlear Implant Users. www.bcig.org

Binzer SM (2000) Self-assessment with the communication profile for the hearing impaired: pre- and post-cochlear implantation. Journal of the Academy of Rehabilitative Audiology 33: 91–114

Blamey P, Arndt P, Bergeron F, Bredberg G, Brimacombe J, Facer G, Larky J, Lindström B, Nedzelski J, Peterson A, Shipp D, Staller S (1996) Factors affecting auditory performance of postlingually deaf adults using cochlear implants. Audiology and Neuro-otology 1: 293–306.

Chen JM, Shipp D, Abdulaziz A, Ng A, Nedzelski JM (2001) Does choosing the 'worse' ear for cochlear implantation affect outcome? Otology and Neurotology 22: 335–9

Clark GM, O'Loughlin BJ, Rickards FW, Tong YC, Williams AJ (1977) The clinical assessment of cochlear implant patients. Journal of Laryngology and Otology 91: 697–708

Cochlear Ltd (2004) Cochlear Implants for Adults – Guidelines for referral to a cochlear implant clinic. Sydney: Cochlear Ltd.

Cullington HE (ed.) (2002) Cochlear Implants: Objective measures. London: Whurr Publishers

Demorest ME, Erdman SA (1987) Development of the communication profile for the hearing impaired. Journal of Speech and Hearing Disorders 52: 129–43

Dowell RC, Brown AM, Mecklenberg DF (1990) Clinical assessment of implanted deaf adults. In: Clark GJ, Tong YC, Patrick JF (eds), Cochlear Prostheses. Edinburgh: Churchill Livingstone

Dowell RC, Hollow R, Winton E, Krauze K, Winfield E (2002) Outcomes for adults using cochlear implants: rethinking selection criteria. Paper presented at the 7th International Cochlear Implant Conference, Manchester, UK, 4–6 September 2002

Erber NP (1988) Communication Therapy for Hearing-impaired Adults. Abbotsford: Clavis

Gailey L (2000) Peer led support groups. Paper presented at 3rd International Symposium on Electronic Implants in Otology and Conventional Hearing Aids. Birmingham, UK, 31 May–2 June 2000.

Gantz BJ, Tyler RS, Knutson JF et al. (1988) Evaluation of five different cochlear implant designs: audiologic assessment and predictors of performance. Laryngoscope 98: 1100–6.

Gfeller K, Turner C, Mehr M, Woodworth G, Fearn R, Knutson J, Witt S, Stordahl J (2002) Recognition of familiar melodies by adult cochlear implant recipients and normal hearing adults. Cochlear Implants International 3: 29–53

Gibson WPR (1992) The effect of electrical stimulation and cochlear implantation on tinnitus. In: Arran JM, Dauman R (eds), Proceedings of the IVth International Tinnitus Seminar, Bordeaux. Amsterdam, Kugler and Ghendini, pp. 403–8.

Gibson WPR (2003) Pre-operative medical and electrophysiological evaluation. Deciphering the cochlear implant test battery workshop. Paper presented at Sydney 10–11 April 2003

Hawthorne G, Hogan A (2002) Measuring disability-specific patient benefit in cochlear implant programs: developing a short form of the Glasgow Health Status Inventory, the Hearing Participation Scale. International Journal Audiology 41: 535–44.

Hazell JWP, Meerton LJ, Conway JJ (1989) Electrical tinnitus suppression (ETS) with a single channel cochlear implant. Journal of Laryngology and Otology 18: 39–44

Hogan A (2001) Hearing Rehabilitation for Deafened Adults: A psychosocial approach. London: Whurr Publishers, 96–114

Hogan A, Taylor A, Code C, (1999) Employment outcomes for people with cochlear implants. Australian Journal of Rehabilitative Counselling 5: 1–8.

Hogan A, Stewart, M, Giles, E (2002) It's a whole new ball game! Employment experiences of people with a cochlear implant. Cochlear Implants International 3: 54–67.

Kawashima T, Iwaki T, Yamamoto K, Doi K, Kudo T (1998). Predictive factors for speech perception in patients with cochlear implants. Journal of Oto-Rhino-Laryngological Society of Japan 101: 829-35

Knutson JF, Hinrichs JV, Tyler RS, Gantz BJ, Schartz HA, Woodword G (1991) Psychological predictors of audiological outcomes of multichannel cochlear implants: preliminary findings. Annals of Otology, Rhinology and Laryngology 100: 817-22

Kuo SCL, Gibson WPR (2002) The role of the promontory stimulation test in cochlear implantation. Cochlear Implants International 3: 19-28

McKenna L (1991) The assessment of psychological variables in cochlear implant patients. In: Cooper H (ed.), Cochlear Implants: A practical Guide. London: Whurr Publishers, 125-145

Muller J, Schon F, Helms J (2002) Speech understanding in Quiet and noise in bilateral users of the MED-EL COMBI 40/40+ cochlear implant system. Ear and Hearing 23: 198-206

Parkin JL, Stewart BE, Danowski K, Haas LJ (1989) Prognosticating speech performance in multichannel cochlear implant patients. Otolaryngology Head and Neck Surgery 101: 314-19.

Psarros C, Incerti P, Abrahams Y, Smither J, Haddon A, Pearce C, Bray M, Gibson WPR, Sanli H, Purdy S, Dawson PW (2002) The role of objective measures for setting initial maps in children: Is it time to get rid of the audiologist? Paper presented at 7th International Cochlear Implant Conference. Manchester, UK, September 2002

Rea PA, Gibson WPR (2003) Evidence for surviving outer hair cell function in congenitally deaf ears. Laryngoscope 113: 2030-4

Robinson K, Gatehouse S, Browning GG (1996) Measuring patient benefit from otorhinolaryngological surgery and therapy. Annals of Otorhinolaryngology 105: 415-22

Rushbrooke E, Pedley K (2002) Outcomes for Congenitally Deafened Adults with Cochlear Implants. Paper presented at XXVIth International Congress of Audiology, Melbourne, Australia, 19 March 2002

Shipp DB, Nedzelski JM (1995) Prognostic indicators of speech recognition performance in adult cochlear implant users: a prospective analysis. Annals of Otology, Rhinology and Laryngology, Supplement 116: 196-206.

Spraggs PD, Burton MJ, Graham JM (1994) Nonorganic hearing loss in cochlear implant candidates. American Journal of Otology 15: 652-7

Summerfield AQ, Marshall DH (1995) Cochlear Implantation in the UK 1990-1994. Main Report. London: HMSO, 91-3

Tucci DL, Niparko JK (2000) Medical and surgical aspects of cochlear implantation. In: Niparko JK (ed.), Cochlear Implants: Principles and practices. Philadelphia: Lippincott Williams & Wilkins.

Van Dijk JE, van Olphen AF, Langereis MC, Mens LHM, Brokx JPL, Smoorenburg GF (1999) Predictors of cochlear implant performance. Audiology 38: 109-16.

Verschuur C, Lutman M (2003) Auditory localization abilities in bilateral cochlear implant recipients using the Nucleus 24 cochlear implant. Cochlear Implants International, 4 (supplement 1): 13-14.

Wechlser D (1997) Wechsler Adult Intelligence Scale, 3rd revision. San Antonio, TX: Psychological Corp.

Winton L, Hollow R, Hill K, Tselepis V (2002) Speech perception selection criteria: who is an implant candidate now? Paper presented at the XXVIth International Congress of Audiology, Melbourne, Australia, 17-21 March 2002

Chapter 3
The 'switch-on' period

KAREN PEDLEY AND ELLEN GILES

The focus of this chapter is on the counselling and support provided during the initial 'switch-on' period of the cochlear implant as the patient adjusts to the sound sensations produced when the auditory nerve is stimulated in a new way. At this early stage, normal conversational level speech can be detected but not necessarily understood. Issues related to device programming or 'mapping' (see p. 55) are covered in general terms only and the reader is referred to the manufacturer's technical manual for greater detail.

As described in Chapter 2, the patient will have been assessed against a variety of medical and audiological criteria. The expectations of the patient and family will have been carefully examined and the possible outcomes of cochlear implantation discussed in detail. The patient and the implant team will have weighed the likely outcomes of implantation against possible alternatives and have decided to proceed to implantation.

The cochlear implant hardware comprises externally worn and internal (surgically implanted) components. The microphone of the speech processor receives sound. The speech processor (either body-worn or ear-level style) analyses and digitizes the sound into coded signals, which are then sent to a transmitter coil. The coil sends the coded signals to the implant where they are converted to electrical signals and sent to the electrode array in the cochlea, usually within the scala tympani. The auditory nerve fibres are thus stimulated and signals are sent to the brain.

Cochlear implant surgery is now an established procedure lasting 60–90 minutes. For the patient and the patient's family, the period around the surgery can be an anxious time. There may be concerns about discomfort or possible, albeit rare, side effects such as dizziness and tinnitus. Some patients find the hospital stay itself quite stressful and many appreciate an inpatient visit from their therapist with whom they already have a rapport. For those patients in whom the better ear is implanted, there is the additional stress of not being able to use the hearing aid in this ear in the period between surgery and the implant being activated. Patients report many intense feelings during this period including isolation, frustration particularly at their increased dependence on others, fear (that the outcome will not meet their own or their family's expectations), excitement and impatience. The family may be required to cope with a 'roller-coaster' of emotions as well as the increased barrier to communication. It is important to discuss these issues with the whole family before surgery.

Patient preparation for switch-on

Once the surgery is over, the patient becomes much more interested in the next stage – 'switch-on' – the process of activating the implanted device described in more detail below. Switch-on takes place between 2 and 6 weeks after surgery, depending on the time taken for the incision to heal. The therapist's goal is to provide a comfortable sound level with the best possible representation of speech. Creating a relaxed, organized and supportive environment, in which the patient remains the focus of attention, helps to reduce anxiety and encourages reliable responses from the patient. Obtaining accurate psychophysical measures depends not only on the therapist's skill and experience, but also on an attentive, focused and well-instructed patient, the patient's concentration, ability to learn new skills and other variables such as fatigue, and if the patient has experienced long periods with no sound input. A good first impression of sound from the implant helps to ensure continued cooperation, interest and compliance by the patient.

Main components of the switch-on

- The external components of the headset and speech processor are fitted and comfort adjustments are made, where necessary.
- The electrodes are systematically activated and the 'threshold' (T) and 'comfort' (C) level of each activated electrode are psychophysically determined. The T level is the current level at which the patient is first clearly able to detect stimulation on that electrode. The C level is the current level that provides a loud stimulus that would be comfortable for several minutes. The current T and C levels for the electrodes are known as the MAP. The difference between these two levels is the dynamic range. During the creation of the MAP, the patient usually hears only the sound created by electrically stimulating one electrode by the computer. The measured T and C levels vary between electrodes and between patients.

- The stimulation provided by the MAP is tested with the therapist's voice by simultaneously activating all of the mapped electrodes. At this point the implant receives input from the environment via the microphone. This provides the patient with an initial impression of electrically stimulated sound.
- The patient learns the practical aspects of managing the external components, particularly fitting the headset, operating the processor controls, managing the batteries, and basic care and maintenance.
- The therapist introduces the patient and support person(s) to communication strategies, which will be developed over the course of the rehabilitation period.

It can save a great deal of time and reduce the potential distractions to clarify practical issues *before the switch-on*. The family should know how long the appointment might last, making allowances for travel arrangements for out-of-town patients. The therapist should ensure that there is enough space and seating for those who will share the switch-on experience. If many people will be involved, a rotation may need to be agreed on beforehand. If the switch-on will be video-recorded, issues such as privacy and access to the tapes can be discussed with the family beforehand.

Unnecessary inconvenience and interruptions to the flow of the appointment can be avoided by providing the patient with an individualized list of items to arrange or bring beforehand such as their spectacles, their own hearing aid where applicable and spare batteries. This serves as a reminder if it will be necessary to trim the hair where the coil attaches, or arrange for alterations to hairstyles, wigs or hairpieces. It is especially important to establish if the patient has any special requirements such as an interpreter, signing or instructions in Braille.

Some patients may be prepared to do 'background reading' in the recuperation period between surgery and switch-on. This can save time at the switch-on by familiarizing the patient with new terminology, providing explanations about the psychophysical processes involved and a framework for the appointment. Given the inherent communication difficulties, any effort to reduce misunderstanding and improve the flow of communication during the appointment is beneficial to all parties. Pre-reading can alleviate some of the anxiety by demystifying the process and increases patient satisfaction by maintaining their involvement and interest at a time when they may feel very isolated.

Patients can be encouraged to read about two areas, mapping and the external hardware. In our clinic we provide:

- A description of the mapping process from the patient's point of view, including what they will hear, examples of what a computer-stimulated electrode can sound like (e.g. beep, buzz, whistle, 'sh') and what responses will be required. It reminds the patient what to expect when he or she hears through the device for the first time. This information can be provided using explanatory notes with diagrams or a subtitled video.
- A description of the speech processor controls, headset and battery management. Either the manufacturer's 'patient handbook' or a short summary with diagrams is provided.

Some patients will use the recuperation time to read personal accounts of switch-on described by cochlear implant (CI) recipients in books or on websites.

In summary, preparation and directed background reading can lead to a less anxious and more focused patient, and free up more time for the therapist to talk with and support the patient through the initial impressions of sound.

Room and equipment set-up

The process of device activation that the patient is about to undergo has been reported by many as one of the major events in his or her life. The patient and the support person have often been through a period of crisis and are now at a turning point. They will look to the therapist to be the lynch pin of this process which is full of unknowns. It helps the patient's sense of security if the therapist and the working environment present as organized and efficient.

The room should be free of distractions, be reasonably quiet, well lit and private, with tissues and drinking water available for the anxious and sometimes tearful patient or family. All the equipment should be tested beforehand, particularly the headset, processor and connections. There is nothing more distressing for the patient than 'false alarms' caused by faulty leads and dead batteries. Faults and problems do sometimes occur and it is advisable to have spares available and on hand, as well as contact numbers for the manufacturer so that any problem can be quickly rectified.

Ideally the seating arrangement will allow the therapist to see both the computer screen on which the mapping is recorded and the patient. The patient's non-verbal cues such as breathing pattern, facial expression and body posture will provide valuable information about the patient's level of interest and concentration, comfort with procedures, impression of sound, energy levels and anxiousness. The patient will find lip-reading easier if the seating arrangement allows close proximity to the therapist and the therapist's face is not in shadow. Some written communication will be necessary because the patient should remove any hearing aid to avoid confusion with sound from the implant, so it is convenient to work across a small bench or table and have pen and paper to hand.

As many of the directions, questions and reassurances are predictable, prompt cards in large typeface can be prepared in advance and save time and effort for both parties. These can include:

- Loudness scale with verbal or visual descriptors.
- Information prompts such as 'First I am going to attach your headset' and 'Please relax while I save the measures we made on the computer!'
- Instruction prompts such as 'Tell me as soon as you hear or feel any sensation or sound' or 'Please tap your finger in time with the sound you hear'.
- Enlarged diagrams of the processor switches.

The therapist will need to consider the position of the video camera, if used, and the family or support person.

Outlining the session

We assume that the patient has been provided with written information beforehand and has had the opportunity to talk with another CI user about his or her experience. The patient should have a broad understanding of how the device will be activated. The therapist can expect the patient to be largely preoccupied with the outcome of the surgery, whether or not the device will 'work' and what speech will sound like. Generally, CI recipients are not interested in lengthy technical explanations and details are not usually recalled well.

As mapping can be a tiring and repetitive process, there is advantage in providing an outline that is visible to everyone showing the order of events. This ensures that nothing is omitted, allows the patient to see how much progress has been made and what lies ahead and so pace him- or herself. A typical outline might be:

- Attaching the headset
- Implant test: testing the electrodes of the implant *in situ*
- Switching on electrodes: creating a MAP
- Introduction to sound: 'live voice' check and adjustment for comfort

- Managing the external components: headset, processor controls, batteries, basic care and maintenance.

Attaching the headset

The surgeon will have checked that the scar from the implant surgery is well healed and free from infection before switch-on. With a transcutaneous link, the therapist adjusts the magnet so that the coil clings and remains in place on the scalp. A magnet force that is too strong may cause skin irritation. Other components such as ear-hook and cord lengths may be adjusted for comfort.

Implant test

The purpose of the implant test is to provide the clinician with diagnostic information about the implant's operation. It can assist the clinician in determining if any electrodes should not be used as a result of the risk of unpleasant auditory or tactile sensations that may be caused by shorts or open circuits. If required, these electrodes can be deactivated. This is particularly useful before switch-on because it can reduce the possibility of an adverse patient reaction to the implant. The facility available for testing the integrity of the implant will depend on which device has been implanted.

It is important to let the patient know the test duration, that they will not hear any sound and that no response is required. The patient will be anxious to learn that all is well and therefore the clinician should provide positive, conservative but not detailed feedback.

Switching on electrodes: creating a MAP

Once the implant test has shown that the device is functioning correctly, the electrodes can be individually activated.

First stimulation

How the patient responds to the first electrically stimulated sounds depends typically on how much residual hearing remains at the time of implant.

In patients with no measurable residual hearing there is a strong desire to experience sound again, particularly in those whose hearing has not been aided or aidable for many years. However, these patients can find it difficult to recognize that they are hearing soft sound, have more difficulty describing the sound, and can take longer to learn to make subjective comparisons of one sound with another. Being without auditory sensation is a deprivation unimaginable to most people and the therapist can expect the patient to be quite emotional when the first sounds are detected. Other reactions that may be observed in this patient group are surprise, startle or alarm, excitement and relief.

In patients who have enough residual hearing to perceive an *auditory* sensation to pure-tone audiometry up to switch-on, the reaction is more concerned with the nature of the percept and how this changes when different electrodes are activated. These patients tend to be more confident and consistent in their responses and more willing and able to describe the auditory percept. However, the therapist should be sensitive to the first reactions. Some may report disappointment that it does not sound more tonal or like a musical note or that it sounds 'fuzzy' or 'harsh'. It is important to reassure the patient that all of their responses are important and avoid any judgemental comments.

Different electrodes in the electrode array stimulate different subpopulations of cochlear neurons. Most implant systems are designed so that basal electrodes stimulate neurons that respond to high-frequency sounds in normal hearing whereas lower frequencies are encoded by stimulating apical electrodes. Patients have described the tones heard during mapping as a 'beep', a 'buzz', a 'chime' and like a 'telephone engaged signal' whereas stimulation of basal electrodes (high frequencies) has been described as a 'whistle' or 'like someone blowing'.

The mapping process can be facilitated if stimulation on the first few electrodes is easy to detect and as pleasant as possible. Electrodes in the middle of the array seem to fulfil these criteria. The basal electrodes may generate a very high-pitched sound sensation that patients may dislike and find difficult to tolerate, and so should be the last to be turned on.

Measuring T levels

As an ascending technique is used with slowly increasing current, patients are warned that it may take a while before they hear the first sound. This ensures that the first sound patients hear is a soft one. Some patients can become concerned if there is an apparent long break in activity, so the sensitive therapist will maintain rapport with the patient.

The patient is given clear instructions such as 'Please tell me when you hear a series of three sounds' and 'Please tap your finger in time with the sound'. It is worth establishing if the patient has any tinnitus that may be confused with the stimulated sound. The patient should be carefully observed because he or she will often move, tap or nod in time with the stimulus before giving any verbal response.

Once the signal on the first electrode has been detected, the level is increased slowly until the patient reports that it is clearly audible. Providing repeated stimulation at this low but clearly audible level allows time for the patient to become accustomed to the sensation. It can increase patient confidence and reinforce the task by starting and stopping the stimulation and asking the patient to indicate the onset and offset of the stimulus. Once the patient is ready to move on, the level of the stimulation is further increased and prompt cards are used to establish the C level.

Measuring the C level

Having heard sounds through the implant for the first time and confirmed that the device is working, the patient begins to relax a little. In spite of this, the therapist should expect most patients to be quite conservative when asked to allow the stimulation to be increased to loud levels. It is important to increase the stimulus level slowly and ensure that the patient is clear about when and how to respond (usually when it is loud but still tolerable for several minutes). The patient is more likely to feel that he or she has *control* of this procedure and to trust the therapist if the therapist reacts quickly to the patient's responses. Trust is a significant issue here because a nervous patient is likely to be too conservative and set C levels too low. The risk is that the patient's initial impression of speech will be poor and negative attitudes may be established.

Patients interpret concepts and learn new tasks in different ways. Some patients respond to written descriptions whereas others work better when the information is presented visually. Being aware of the patient's strengths and weaknesses is one area where information from the assessment by the implant team psychologist can assist in the rehabilitation. Training patients to give appropriate C levels can be achieved by asking the patient to track along a horizontal loudness scale with loudness descriptors, or a custom-made loudness scale using the patient's own descriptors. Some patients prefer a visual representation; others use a hand signal or sign language.

Any descriptive scale with a *continuum* is preferable on the first day because it is important to know when a moderate loudness level has been reached. The nature of the loudness growth function for electrical stimulation means that the perception of loudness can increase rapidly once it reaches 'moderately loud' level. Consequently, smaller stimulus current step sizes may be appropriate. If the patient is still very nervous with the louder stimulus, use of a *patient-controlled* stimulus knob can help. The patient's first estimate of comfortable loudness judgement may be later refined after further exposure to electrical stimulation.

The ultimate aim of an accurately measured dynamic range from T to C levels is to place the whole critical speech spectrum within the useful dynamic range of the CI.

How many electrodes at switch-on?

The guidelines of the manufacturer should be followed for switch-on. However, with postlingually deafened adults, it is generally preferable to switch all electrodes on with approximate T levels to give a fuller representation of sound than to turn on fewer electrodes with very accurate thresholds. On the first day, however, it is recommended to re-test the first few T levels because these may change quite significantly as a result of familiarity with the stimulus, procedures and practice effect.

If the patient has been accustomed to a predominantly low-frequency stimulus from a hearing aid for a long time, the sound from the implant will seem relatively high pitched. If the patient describes the sound as unacceptably 'screechy' or 'whiney', the sound of speech can be made more acceptable by leaving the most basal electrodes off initially. As the patient gains experience with the implant, those electrodes producing the higher pitch percept can be gradually switched on.

The other factor to balance when deciding the number of electrodes to activate in the first session is the patient's concentration. The patient will invest a great deal of effort and attention to detect the threshold level stimuli and this, together with the high level of arousal, stress, exhilaration and emotion, can leave the patient drained. Maintaining rapport with the patient, e.g. by periodically advising him or her how many electrodes have been activated, monitoring the repeatability of responses and watching the body language, will enable the therapist to stop before the patient is too fatigued and leave some mental energy for learning to handle the device. The increased use of interpolation of T and C levels from adjacent electrodes in manufacturer's software is making this aspect much quicker and easier.

Balancing

Once sufficient electrodes have been activated to create a MAP, adjacent electrode pairs or triplets are balanced for loudness. This important psychoacoustical procedure requires the patient to compare and evaluate the relative loudness of electrodes that may produce a different pitch sensation. If a MAP is not balanced, part of the speech signal may appear too loud or be inaudible, creating an impression of 'fading in and out' or 'popping'.

Although the concept of balancing the loudness of sounds of different pitch will be a difficult one for a new CI recipient, if it is performed in each session it becomes an integral part of the mapping process, so skill level quickly increases and a better MAP is produced. Analogies such as a piano keyboard to explain the different pitches can be useful. The importance of balancing for improving the 'naturalness', 'smoothness', quality and intelligibility of speech needs to be explained to the patient.

Introduction to sound: going 'live'

'Going live' means that the MAP is loaded on to the speech processor and all of the electrodes are activated. The patient hears sound from the environment.

Before the device is finally switched on the patient is again reminded that it will not sound like a hearing aid. Patients should be warned that it may sound artificial and possibly unpleasant for the first few days and that they are likely to hear speech but not necessarily understand it.

All of the programmed electrodes are now turned on and the therapist should face the patient and speak at a soft-to-medium level to judge the first impression. When the CI recipient begins to speak, he or she often falters, because the feedback is unfamiliar. The patient is reassured that this is quite normal.

The therapist now begins the process of easing the patient through the initial reaction to sound and orienting the CI recipient to the relationship between the CI sound and its acoustic origin. The therapist may use familiar phrases, general conversation and family voices, as well as providing examples of common environmental sounds to explore the patient's reactions further. Examples are paper rustling, cup and spoon, knocking at the door, light switch, running tap water, coughing, door closing, rubbing the hands together, a zipper, closing a drawer, keys jangling and humming a well-known tune. Any support people present should be reminded to talk in a normal level voice with normal steady rhythm and to face the CI recipient. The descriptions of speech through the implant on the first day are very varied. Examples are 'like talking with your ears under water', 'like a radio off-station', 'robotic', 'like talking with your hand in front of your mouth' and 'like a dog barking'.

Some common patient reactions to switch on are:

* surprise at hearing own voice
* relief
* amazement
* disappointment at initial voice quality
* laughter
* feeling overwhelmed.

The 'live' test should allow sufficient time for the patient to begin adjustment to the sensation of sound in a supportive and controlled environment and have any questions or concerns addressed by the therapist. In this context support means that, as part of the settling process, the patient is provided with the opportunity to express how he or she is feeling about the switch-on. The therapist acknowledges and legitimizes any reactions that the patient may have (e.g. disappointment). Support engenders a sense of open acceptance – that one allows the reactions to be 'tabled' as it were. The problems stated do not have to be resolved, but timely words of understanding ('many patients have reacted in this way when the device is first switched on') and encouragement ('it may take a while before you can make sense of what you are hearing presently') may be helpful.

The therapist now checks, and demonstrates to the patient, that he or she is able to detect a range of speech sounds at conversational levels in the audition-alone condition. The Ling five-sound test may be used (Ling, 1990). These sounds are 'ah' as in hard, 'ee' as in feet, 'oo' as in food, 'sh' as in ship and 's' as in soft. Clinics may add other sounds to adapt the test for local speech characteristics, e.g. in Australia, some clinics add the back vowel 'or', because 'oo' is not a back vowel in Australian speech. Also 'mm', as in most, may be included for better coverage of the detection of low frequencies (Romanik, 1990). The patient may be asked to indicate, by raising a hand, if the sounds are audible (but the therapist should not insist on correct imitation at this stage). In the majority of adult CI recipients there is 100% detection on this simple task, with the exception that the unforced 's' sound may not be detected if insufficient basal electrodes have been activated. Patients with significant residual hearing and recent hearing aid experience before implantation may be able to imitate all of these sounds.

At this point the patient may be asked to perform a simple discrimination task because it is important that the patient is achieving as early as possible. This is more important with patients who have had no, or minimal, aidable hearing before implantation, e.g. the patient may be asked to discriminate between their own name and the name(s) of a family member with different (and, if possible, highly contrasting) syllable number. The names can be written down and identified as they are spoken. The CI recipient is asked to discriminate which name is spoken. Lip-reading may be used initially. Alternatively, the therapist may demonstrate the highly contrasting sounds 'aa' and 'sh' while the patient watches the electrode light display of the computer interface unit. This device shows which electrodes are being stimulated by the sound. The patient can be asked to indicate which of the two sounds was heard by pointing to one of two cards, 'aa' and 'sh'. This can be done with, and without, the aid of the light display. Other simple tasks may be to count the number of times the therapist taps on the table, to discriminate between their spoken name and an environmental sound such as tearing paper, or to discriminate two highly contrasting environmental sounds such as pouring water and tapping a spoon on a cup.

As the patient has set the maximum output of each electrode, loud stimuli should be comfortable. However, this should always be verified because loudness summation can occur when all the electrodes are activated simultaneously. This means that the perception of loudness of all of the electrodes is greater than the loudness perception of sound from individual electrodes. The therapist's voice level should be gradually increased and the patient should be asked to indicate if the sound exceeds a comfortable level. Some patients' reactions to loud stimuli may be very conservative if they have had no recent exposure to sound. Other loud stimuli that can be used include cup and spoon, running water, cellophane and handclap. In most programming systems, it is possible to change the parameters of the MAP in various ways to improve the patient's perception of sound further.

The patient and family can be reassured of various positive outcomes already evident including:

- The ability to respond to *soft* sound – this can be further demonstrated with tissue paper at arm's length or a soft tap on the desk.
- The ability of the patient to hear and monitor his or her own voice. Family members may comment on the reduction in voice level and some vocal quality changes may be immediately obvious in some cases. The patient is reassured that the sound of the voice will improve as the MAP is fine-tuned and as they grow more accustomed to hearing all of the frequency components.
- The patient's spontaneous response such as turning to look for the source of sounds in the room. Examples may be detecting a family member's voice from behind or awareness of the computer fans.

Managing the external components

The remainder of the appointment is used for the practical issues such as:
- Practise attaching the headset
- How to wear the processor, especially management of cables where applicable (see Chapter 11 for suggestions)
- Using the speech processor controls
- Battery issues including battery life and factors that reduce it, recharging, managing intermittency, appropriate battery types and audible battery warnings

- An introduction to care and maintenance of the equipment should be given including keeping the equipment dry, cleaning battery contacts, etc.

Detailed practical issues are not discussed here, because they will be specific to the implant system fitted.

The next section describes the therapist's goals for the period after switch-on, and how the family can support the CI recipient during this period. Some of the questions most frequently asked by CI recipients are discussed.

Coping with the first few days: the patient's perspective

Another milestone has been reached, the implant has been activated and the CI recipient now focuses on the quality of the sound through the implant. In the next few weeks he or she will gradually be reintroduced to the world of sound. After the excitement of the first few days and the relief that the device is functioning, the patient may experience disappointment as he or she realizes the limitations of the device. The therapist has a number of objectives at this point:

- The CI recipient will re-learn how to *listen and attend* to auditory stimuli.
- The CI recipient will become increasingly *tolerant* to sound.
- The CI recipient will increasingly accept the way that speech sounds. Despite the repeated counselling that speech will not sound as he or she remembers it, and verbal acceptance of this *expectation*, it is human nature to *hope* that speech will sound like memory of speech. From now on the CI recipient is confronted with the reality on a daily basis and must find some personal level of *acceptance*.
- The CI recipient will gradually learn about the implant's *advantages and limitations.*

It can help patients to remain motivated during this period if they feel that they are continually achieving. Both the therapist and the support person play an important support role in providing feedback. One of the patient's greatest needs is to be reassured that the implant was the correct decision. The therapist and the patient's family can help by pointing out when the patient responds to sounds that he or she could not hear previously. Some examples are:

- When the CI recipient detects a soft sound, such as a light switch
- When the CI recipient responds to his or her name without visual cues

- When the CI recipient responds to a sound outside the room, such as a voice or the office telephone
- That his or her voice level drops as soon as the processor is turned on
- When the CI recipient turns readily to acknowledge a new speaker.

Family members can help by drawing the CI recipient's attention to positive changes that occur at home such as if he or she:

- rarely interrupts the speaker during a conversation
- places kitchen utensils down with considerably less noise
- notices and acknowledges when someone enters the room unseen
- makes fewer idiosyncratic sounds between utterances such as sighs, groans
- eats more quietly
- converses for longer periods without fatigue
- does not lean forwards and/or frown when listening
- smiles more or generally appears more relaxed.

It can be helpful to remind the CI recipient that repeated exposure to sound stimuli leads to some being 'filtered out' as irrelevant or unimportant whereas other more relevant sounds will continue to command the attention. The implication of this is that, until the patient becomes used to hearing new background noises, she or he will be *conscious* of much more sound than previously, which is often tiring. Periods of time out can help the adjustment. It is for this reason that it may be recommended to the CI recipient that he or she experience and become accustomed to quiet environments and one or two speakers before facing the challenge of large groups and unfamiliar or noisy environments.

Each CI recipient will respond to his or her new world of sound in a unique way. However, there are a few questions and issues that most CI recipients ask about or wish to discuss.

'How many hours should I wear it?'

Patients' abilities to cope with the increased amount of auditory information can depend on the amount of exposure to auditory stimulation before switch-on, the range of frequencies to which they are accustomed, how they cope with change and their general level of tolerance for 'noise' (i.e. sound that they are not attending to). Those who have heard very little sound from hearing aids for months or years find a few hours each day in sessions of 2–3 hours manageable initially. Patients with more recent loss, more residual hearing and/or who have been wearing hearing aids in the non-implanted ear right up to switch-on may report being able to wear it all day long immediately.

'Should I continue to use lip-reading?'

Encourage the CI recipient to listen AND watch. Being used to receiving most of the information visually, the addition of sound can be distracting initially. Some CI recipients who were implanted with no measurable hearing talk about the sound 'lagging behind' the lip-read signal. As they become more proficient in processing the sound of speech, they report that the two signals appear to become more synchronized.

'Should I wear my hearing aid in the non-implanted ear?

Many CI recipients with aidable hearing in the ear contralateral to the implant have learned to integrate signals from the hearing aid and cochlear implant successfully in spite of reporting different quality from each side. The benefits of bimodal fittings reported by our patients include increased awareness of sound from the non-implanted side and better speech understanding in noise when wearing both devices. Tyler et al. (2002) reported cases of improved localization ability when both devices were worn. However, it was suggested that the relative levels of performance from the two devices could compromise binaural integration. Studies in children and adults (Ching et al., 2001, 2002) have shown that, on average, there are significant binaural advantages in speech perception tests, localization and everyday communication (e.g. identifying a speaker in a group) when an adjusted hearing aid is worn with the implant compared with a cochlear implant alone. In this study, loudness balancing between the hearing aid and the cochlear implant was performed. No binaural interference effects were measured.

The decision to continue to wear the hearing aid should be made on an individual basis and may depend on several factors such as the residual speech perception with the aid alone, how well the patient likes and tolerates the aided sound, how well the patient initially performs with the implant alone and practical concerns (see Chapter 11). In our experience, wearing *only* the implant for several hours a day in the initial stages allows the patient to focus on the sound from the implant and may accelerate the speed at which a CI recipient learns to use the new information. For this reason, it is important that auditory and communication training in the clinic and at home is performed with the implant alone (see Chapter 4). Some patients report that they use the hearing aid (either with or without the implant) whenever tired or stressed or when they need help to recognize a sound. A new CI recipient may find it helpful to wear the implant in quiet situations, but wear both devices in more challenging environments. Some centres encourage patients to wear an aid on the non-implanted side to maintain stimulation of the auditory pathways. This may have some advantage if this ear is later implanted.

'What can I do to improve understanding?'

The CI recipient should be reminded of basic communication strategies such as reducing distance to the speaker, optimizing the lighting, arranging seating so that the speaker faces him or her, or is on the implanted side and reducing the ambient noise.

'What can I do to learn to identify background sounds?'

Use of an environmental sounds checklist (Plant, 1984) can provide a starting point. Initially, the focus may be on developing an awareness of the gross differences between common environmental sounds. The patient could be asked to note when each sound has been heard and/or recognized. Some CI recipients enjoy systematically making the sounds on the list for themselves. The patient should be aware of the potential for family members to facilitate the identification process by labelling sounds as they arise. Some patients have found tapes of environmental sounds helpful.

'How will I cope with background noise?'

The CI recipient is encouraged to wear the processor in quiet environments initially. Soon after switch-on the patient should know how to use any noise-reduction facilities and volume or sensitivity control on the speech processor. A lapel microphone can be particularly effective in improving the signal-to-noise ratio in group situations or in public places. The CI recipient should be aware of how to connect it and different ways to use it. This is covered in more detail in Chapter 11.

As some CI recipients can quickly become distressed, even overwhelmed by loud unfamiliar noise, it may be advisable to leave the implant off in traffic, shopping centres and planes, for example, in the first few days. Some patients prefer to turn the processor down when first travelling in a car. The patient may need to be reminded of environmental noise management *strategies* (see Chapter 7) such as closing doors and windows, and use of tablecloths and rugs, because the CI recipient is now potentially capable of detecting more environmental stimuli.

'When can I wear my speech processor at work?'

There are a number of different factors to consider including noise levels, safety factors, support at work, and patient and employer expectations.

If it is a very noisy occupation, the CI recipient may be better to leave the processor off at work initially and then gradually introduce it at lower stimulus level, e.g. reduced volume or sensitivity setting. If there are safety issues, such as the risk of not hearing a forklift truck, the implant should be introduced at work as soon as possible.

CI users in quiet occupations, such as office work, may successfully wear their processor at work soon after switch-on. Strategies to reduce noise can expedite a CI recipient's return to work. The patient and/or employer can consider such measures as situating the CI recipient's desk away from printers, fax machines, doorways and corridors. In an open plan office, divider panels can provide some noise attenuation.

It can assist a CI recipient's return to work after implant if the supervisor and/or work colleagues are supportive and understand the following points. The CI recipient is learning to adjust to and identify background sounds, still requires visual cues, may be made tired by the additional sound initially and needs time to respond to speech through the implant. Ideally, work colleagues should understand the limitations of the implant, such as limited microphone directionality and hearing over distance in meetings. Some employers will accept a phased return to the workplace that may allow a CI recipient to return to work sooner.

Whenever the CI recipient returns to work, the expectations of both the patient and the employer must reflect the CI recipient's *current* experience with the device and ability to understand speech. This is particularly important with regard to more challenging aspects of hearing at work such as telephone use and hearing in meetings.

Other questions from the CI recipient usually relate to practical issues such as magnet tightness, wearing of spectacles with the processor microphone, water damage, cable management, insurance of the external components, basic troubleshooting, and how to access a 'loaner device' from the clinic in case of apparent breakdown.

Counselling the family in the switch-on period

The family members can often be very tired at this appointment. A great deal of energy has been expended to get the CI recipient to this point. The family frequently accompany and support the CI recipient through the assessment appointments, make phone calls and arrangements on his or her behalf, changing their own schedules and putting their own needs aside to cope with the added responsibilities. At the same time they cope daily with the communication difficulties. Now for the first time many of them start to 'let go'.

It is worth reiterating that the CI recipient will hear but not necessarily understand speech and that this is caused by his or her inexperience with the electrical representation of speech rather than its inaudibility. The family can be encouraged to use normal speech levels, face the CI recipient, be patient and resist the temptation to 'test' the CI user by covering their mouth, because this is likely to lead to frustration on the part of the patient. To assist with the process of introducing the family and significant others to better communication strategies, a list of suggestions is given below.

After living with a severely deafened person, some support people may have developed communication habits over long periods of time that will be inappropriate for a CI recipient, e.g. a loud voice, exaggerated facial features, leaning over to talk directly into the person's ear or chunking the sentence into two or three parts which removes context cues. The therapist can tactfully help them to self-monitor such behaviour and replace them with other strategies more appropriate for a CI recipient.

Although the support person may not be able to cope with a lot of new information all at once, the therapist can aim to cover suggestions in the following areas over the first few days.

Helping the CI recipient to cope with the new auditory environment

Overall sound level

The need to reduce the overall sound at home may seem obvious to the therapist. However, the family have been accustomed to living with a very hearing-impaired person who could not even *detect* many soft or even moderate level sounds. It is important that they now appreciate the CI recipient's ability to hear all levels of sound. This can be demonstrated in the clinic using, for example, the rustle of tissue paper, turning the pages of a book, footsteps on the carpet, the chink of two glasses knocking together, rubbing fingers against clothing, opening the tap or a zipper, closing the door, drawing the curtains and using a light switch. The family may be as surprised as the patient by the number and variety of sounds that the CI recipient is now able to detect. Suggestions to reduce unnecessary noise could include closing doors to reduce sound from noisy electrical appliances and turning off the radio or TV when conversation is taking place. Such measures can reduce the number of distractions and lessen the possibility of 'overwhelming' the CI recipient, leading to stress and fatigue.

Identification of background sounds

Being able to hear, but not identify, sound can be a disconcerting and sometimes alarming experience for the CI recipient, e.g. a CI recipient described an experience of being in the elevator of a department store with her mother. 'I could hear a man's voice speaking, but there was no-one else in the lift.' Her mother explained that the voice was a recorded announcement at each floor – something that the CI recipient was hitherto unaware of. The family or support person plays an important role in the first few days, labelling sounds such as the phone ringing, particularly in a high context situation, e.g. demonstrating the doorbell. As a sound may be quite unlike the hearing aid version, it may need to be identified several times before it is learned.

In our experience most patients learn to identify common environmental sounds within the first month, although the repertoire continues to grow during the first year. Patients may learn to use any light/visual displays on the processor to indicate the *presence* of sound. With increasing miniaturization, however, these visual cues will not always be available and the support person will be even more important.

Family gatherings

It is understandable that family and friends will be anxious to visit the CI recipient soon after switch-on to learn about the new auditory experience. Unfortunately this creates a difficult listening situation for the new CI recipient who does not have the experience to extract speech cues from the overall background noise level generated from a gathering of people, even with the dedicated processor settings for noise reduction. The family should be counselled to keep numbers small where possible, talk one at a time, and allow the CI recipient the opportunity to talk one-on-one away from the main group and to have quiet periods of 'time out'.

Awareness of specific features of some cochlear implant systems

There are a number of features of implant systems that the family or support people should understand. If used correctly, they can be used to advantage rather than hindering communication. The following are the features that have implications for the communication style of the family.

The directional microphone

It can be demonstrated by walking around the CI recipient that the microphone is more sensitive to sound from the front than from the sides or behind.

The external components usually comprise *one* microphone worn over the pinna. This means that the head can act as a baffle for high-frequency components of speech coming from the non-implanted side. This leads to speech being degraded and sounding 'muffled'. Family members can be encouraged to sit on the implanted side or directly facing the CI recipient.

The CI recipient-mapped threshold and comfort levels

These ensure that conversation level speech is both *audible* and comfortable. Therefore, in most circumstances, there is no advantage in raising the voice. It is important to use the voice consistently, i.e. not to mouth words.

Lapel microphone

The external 'clip-on' or 'lapel' microphone can be plugged into the processor to assist communication whenever facing the CI recipient is not possible, such as in a car. This increases the level of speech relative to the surrounding noise.

The communication needs of an inexperienced CI recipient

An inexperienced CI recipient gradually learns to associate the sounds from the implant with the prior knowledge of speech sounds. The 'de-coding' takes time, experience and repeated exposure to speech. CI recipients often comment that they most enjoy talking to people who take their time, separate their words, and speak clearly and steadily. There are many communication strategies that the family can be encouraged to use. The list below provides some initial pointers:

- The CI recipient may be highly dependent on lip-reading initially so *capture their attention* before speaking.
- *Remain facing* the CI recipient and keep the head reasonably still – the CI recipient will need to confirm what he or she hears with the familiar visual signal.
- *Speak steadily*, without rushing, so that the CI recipient can hear each word. It is equally important to counsel against slowing the speech down in an exaggerated fashion.
- *Do not shout* – this is likely to result in a distorted or even uncomfortable signal.
- Allow the CI recipient plenty of *time to respond* because with limited experience it takes more time to de-code the information.
- Provide *topic clues* whenever there is a change of subject in conversation. This allows the CI recipient to predict some words and to use context to fill in the gaps whenever the sentence is incompletely heard.

- Speak in relatively *short sentences* to reduce the demand on auditory memory.
- Encourage family members to use the redundancy in speech by *rephrasing* the same sentence.
- Use more common *'everyday' words and phrases* because these are more likely to be understood.
- Some names or unusual words may need to be *written* down.

Helping the CI recipient to adjust the voice level

With the improved auditory feedback, the CI recipient's voice can change from a loud, harsh, wildly fluctuating and somewhat nasal sounding voice to a more natural and better-regulated one. This is one of the greatest sources of pleasure for the support person. However, after periods of silence or in background noise, the CI recipient's voice may increase in level again. The family can assist with voice training in conjunction with positive feedback by:

- Demonstrating a soft, medium and loud voice to the CI recipient, perhaps by reading a sentence or short passage. This allows the CI recipient to experience the auditory sensation created by differing levels of loudness.
- Listening to the CI recipient read a passage and providing feedback on voice level. Adding background noise so that the CI recipient may learn compensatory adjustments can extend this skill.
- Developing a system of discrete cues that can be used outside the home to guide the patient to an appropriate voice level.

Coping with tinnitus

The effects of the cochlear implant on pre-existing tinnitus are variable; the tinnitus may remain the same, become less noticeable or (more rarely) be exaggerated by use of a cochlear implant. Several studies have reported mixed outcomes for patients with pre-existing tinnitus. In some cases, unilateral implantation resulted in bilateral tinnitus suppression (McKerrow et al., 1991). Tyler (1995) reported the outcomes of 82 adult patients who received the 3M/Vienna single-channel device, the multi-channel Nucleus or the Ineraid cochlear implant after 24 months of implant use. Twenty-two patients had reported 'bothersome tinnitus' preoperatively; 2 of the 22 patients (9%) showed an increase in their tinnitus after 24 months of implant use. However, 41% of patients in this study showed a decrease in their tinnitus handicap of more than 10%. These figures are similar to those reported by Thedinger et al. (1985) who suggest that around half of the patients gain significant tinnitus reduction whereas less than 8% report that tinnitus is worse.

Rarely, cochlear implantation may produce tinnitus in a patient who did not experience this symptom preoperatively.

The importance of counselling the patient about the range of outcomes cannot be overstressed. The following suggestions may help the patient to keep any tinnitus manageable and reduce any detrimental effect on the psychophysical measures made at mapping:

- If a patient's tinnitus has been problematic pre-implant, it is worth warning him or her that it may be exacerbated for a few days at switch-on time.
- Reassure the CI recipient that in most cases the tinnitus becomes less noticeable. In our experience, this occurs over the first few weeks.
- Use a series of at least two beeps when mapping to avoid confusion with the tinnitus, especially at very soft sensation levels.
- Counsel against over-setting C levels as a way of 'masking' the tinnitus.
- Use time out if the sound from the cochlear implant appears to exacerbate tinnitus. Occasionally, a global reduction in C levels may help.
- If the patient notices the tinnitus less when wearing the implant, advise him or her to expect the tinnitus to be more apparent again after the processor is taken off.
- Encourage the patient with persistent tinnitus to use the sound level controls to reduce the perception of their tinnitus rather than to mask it totally with ambient sound.
- Tinnitus can be exacerbated by fatigue and anxiety, both of which are more likely around the switch-on period. Discuss strategies for stress reduction with the patient.

Assistive listening devices

Most implant systems include a variety of add-on devices which are used in conjunction with the speech processor to improve the signal-to-noise ratio. If the switch-on is over 2 or 3 days there is sufficient time to demonstrate each device and outline potential uses. Some patients are very interested in how the TV signal can be fed directly into the speech processor and how to use the telephone. However, many patients will be too preoccupied with the initial sound and managing the processor to attend in any great detail to peripheral equipment at this stage.

As the limitations of the implant become more apparent over the next 3 months, patients become more motivated to experiment with assistive listening devices (ALDs), such a the lapel microphone. Teaching the potential advantages of each device can be accomplished cost-effectively in a group format if patients have enough in common to make sharing of experiences and solutions to problems worthwhile.

When the auditory training has reached the level where the difficulty is increased by introducing background noise or degrading the signal, the improvement in signal-to-noise ratio made possible by the ALDs can be demonstrated. The use of ALDs with cochlear implants is discussed in more detail in Chapter 11.

References

Ching TY, Psarros C, Hill M, Dillon H, Incerti P (2001) Should children who use cochlear implants wear hearing aids in the opposite ear? Ear and Hearing 22: 365–80

Ching TY, Incerti P, Hill M, Brew J, Psarros C (2002) Binaural Benefits for Children and Adults Who use Hearing Aids and Cochlear Implants in Opposite Ears. Sydney: National Acoustic Laboratory Annual Report 2002/2002

Ling D (1990) Foundations of Spoken Language for Hearing Impaired Children. Washington, DC: Alexandra Graham Bell Association for the Deaf

McKerrow WS, Schreiner CS, Snyder RL, Merzenich MM, Toner J G (1991) Tinnitus suppression by cochlear implants. Annals of Otology, Rhinology and Laryngology 100: 552–8

Plant G (1984) COMMTRAM. A Communication Training Program for Profoundly Deaf Adults. Sydney: National Acoustics Laboratories

Romanik S (1990) Auditory Skills Program, Book 1, for Students with Hearing Impairment. New South Wales: Department of School Education

Thedinger B, House WF, Edgerton BJ (1985) Cochlear implants for tinnitus. Annals of Otology, Rhinology and Laryngology 94: 10–13

Tyler RS (1995) Tinnitus in the profoundly hearing-impaired and the effects of cochlear implants. Annals of Otology, Rhinology and Laryngology, Supplement 165, 104(Pt 2): 25–30

Tyler RS, Parkinson AJ, Wilson BS, Witt S, Preece JP, Noble W (2002) Patients utilizing a hearing aid and a cochlear implant: speech perception and localization. Ear and Hearing 23: 98–105

Chapter 4
Aural rehabilitation following cochlear implantation: key objectives of an aural rehabilitation programme

KAREN PEDLEY AND ELLEN GILES

In the first few days after the cochlear implant is switched on, the patient encounters many new auditory experiences. Many self-made sounds such as the patient's voice, coughing, eating and sighing may be heard for the first time in many years. Environmental stimuli, which may or may not be recognized, can be a source of wonder, satisfaction, surprise and irritation. Those frequently commented on are footsteps, running water, bird song, keys jangling, aeroplanes, rain, the telephone ring and the tick of a car indicator. Patients with long-standing hearing loss may discover sounds that they did not know existed, e.g. several of our patients discovered that some elevators have voice announcers, the closing mechanism on a favourite bag actually 'clicked' and that ice-cubes 'cracked' as they melted. For most patients, however, the focus is on the way speech sounds through the implant. In the first few days, descriptions such as 'electronic', 'robotic', 'like someone speaking underwater' and 'screechy' are not uncommon.

The therapist can expect a wide range of abilities among patients at this stage. Some patients may report that all environmental stimuli appear to 'make the same noise'. Others will quickly interpret the stimulus from a source such as paper rustling and recognize it as the sound of turning pages, for example. Post-implant speech perception abilities in the week immediately after device activation vary considerably from patient to patient. A pre- or perilingually deafened adult, or an adult with a long period of auditory deprivation pre-implant, may hear but not recognize *any* words after the first few days. At the other end of the spectrum, a recently deafened adult with some residual speech recognition before implantation may be

73

able to accurately repeat back whole phrases within 24 hours after device activation.

Overview of the post-implant rehabilitation programme

The process of rehabilitation outlined in this and the following two chapters takes the patient from the initial device activation stage to maximizing the patient's individual potential with the implant and ultimately coming to terms with the final outcome. The patient's main preoccupation immediately after switch-on is usually with external device management and the nature of the sound being perceived in broad terms. In the period that follows, the patient focuses more on his or her individual communication needs, specific goals and how the sound from the implant can help him or her to be part of the world again. In particular, patients focus on what is achievable and how quickly it can be achieved. Through the rehabilitation process, the patient will become familiar with both the capabilities and the limitations of the device and the compensatory strategies required to manage those limitations.

The role of the therapist is to:

*   form an appropriate plan of intervention based on the patient's pre-implant goals, the initial level of speech perception and current communication skills
*   provide both general and goal-specific information counselling
*   provide support counselling for the patient and his or her family.

Once achievable goals have been agreed on between the cochlear implant (CI) recipient and therapist (see p. 76), the intervention plan begins with identifying the skills that the patient needs to meet each specific goal. The training required to build these skills can be drawn from two approaches: auditory training and communication therapy. Examples of intervention plans can be found in Chapter 6.

The objective of auditory training in the context of rehabilitation of CI recipients is to maximize the patient's listening skills and ability to learn to relate new sensations provided by electrical stimulation of the cochlea to previously learned auditory patterns. In one aspect of auditory training, the CI recipient practises the perception and recognition of different aspects of speech stimuli from individual speech features such as word stress and intonation, through to phrase, sentence and passage level material. Auditory training may also include guided practice in environmental sound recognition (see Chapter 3) and perception of other non-speech sounds (e.g. telephones tones, music).

A second, but equally important, objective is for the patient to become more conscious of all of the available cues in conversation, i.e. topic, semantic and contextual clues, and to practise using these cues to enhance speech perception. The value of linguistic cues to fill perceptual gaps has been reported elsewhere (Jeffers and Barley, 1971; Hull, 1976; Erber, 1996, 2002). The importance of working with the patient's *existing* linguistic skills rather than expecting (probably unrealistically) to enhance an adult's linguistic level of sophistication has been emphasized (Erber, 1996). Skills in this area can be enhanced through auditory training with synthetic level material (see p. 77) and communication therapy, which provides 'practice in accessing spoken interaction under conditions that mimic . . . elements of everyday speech perception in conversation' (Lind, 2004). Communication therapy develops the patient's and significant others' awareness of, and practical experience with, strategies to enhance the message, the environment in which the conversation takes place, and the CI recipient's and significant others' responses to the various obstacles to free-flowing conversation that may arise.

In our experience, CI recipients benefit from a programme in which auditory training and communication therapy are performed concurrently. This objective is based on the premise that one of patients' primary goals is to maximize their *communication* potential as they seek to remake themselves as participants in the hearing culture of family, social life and, possibly, work (Hogan, 2001). It is generally accepted that everyday speech contains significant redundancy, i.e. the listener does not need to hear the entire communication accurately to understand the message, only correctly to perceive sufficient numbers of key words. Unfortunately, even CI recipients with good speech recognition in quiet will not always understand *sufficient* words to follow the conversation in poor listening conditions. This is caused by the distorted nature of the sound from the implant, together with the signal degradation that may result from environmental factors, the situation and the speaker. A rehabilitation programme that emphasizes only *perceptual* abilities is unlikely adequately to equip the CI recipient to cope in the real world. Empowering the patient to cope in a variety of listening environments may best be achieved when the patient learns skills to *compensate* for the incomplete stimulus and to manage everyday conversational settings better. Teaching compensatory skills early in the rehabilitation programme reinforces the important message that the cochlear implant is not 'normal hearing' – it is an aid to hearing. This approach may also contribute to a positively reinforcing cycle of factors affecting outcome as shown in Figure 4.1. One of the initial goals in our programmes is to encourage the CI recipient to make intensive and extensive use of the device. In our experience, CI recipients who are experiencing frequent successes are positively reinforced to make greater use of the device. Those who wear the device more extensively appear to make progress faster. Especially in the early stages of implant use when the auditory signal may be more degraded, the CI recipient may be more likely to experience some success and feel confident in conversational situations if a range of strategies is at their disposal.

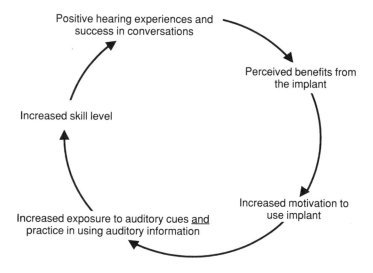

Figure 4.1 Positive cycle of affirmation and skills enhancement.

Aural rehabilitation: a range of service provision

Economic pressures on health services generally mean that there is great diversity in the degree to which programmes include a rehabilitation component. Some authors describe programmes that dedicate regular time for training and rehabilitation ranging from several hours to several days (Cook, 1991; Borsco et al., 1996; Strauss-Schier and Rost, 1996). Other practitioners consider that the quality-of-life improvement with the device alone is so great that rehabilitation is too time-consuming to be justified in terms of perceived costs relative to benefits.

There is also much variation in the range of rehabilitation activities offered. In some centres rehabilitation is limited to advice counselling; others offer regular speech perception training with a therapist. Other programmes again offer sophisticated computer-controlled and -scored auditory visual training exercises (Cook, 1991). Some programmes use role-play to help CI recipients to identify the communication strategies on which they would most benefit from focusing (Eisenwort, 1985; Eisenwort et al., 1996).

Many resources have been developed for CI recipients to use at home. These include recordings of environmental sounds (Cook, 1991) and books on audiotape with written comprehension questions (Tye-Murray et al., 1996). Video laser disc programmes have been employed in one programme to teach conversational repair strategies. They provide immediate feedback, in an auditory–visual mode, of the effect of specific repair strategies (Tye-Murray, 1991; Tye-Murray and Witt, 1997). Patient rehabilitation manuals designed for home use have also been developed at a number of centres (e.g. Eisenwort, 1985). Some contain support and information counselling, communication guidance, tips for the 'support person', auditory training exercises (Pedley, 2000) and sound detection lists (Borsco et al., 1996); others provide CI recipient-administered self-tests (Wayner et al., 1998) and still others include tips on how to improve speech reading and suggestions for incorporating listening into daily life events (Tye-Murray et al., 1996). Some programmes employ an instructional film demonstrating appropriate communication practices for the *families* of CI recipients (Tye-Murray, 1993).

Rehabilitation programmes also vary in relation to who is included in the rehabilitation process. Some programmes involve the patient and therapist only. Others employ activities that specifically include significant others such as family members, neighbours, friends or other support people. These people may be involved both in the clinic and/or through a formal or informal home-training programme (Edgerton, 1985). Some implant programmes report the value of including other CI recipients in the rehabilitation process. This may take the form of an informal group meeting where CI recipients share experiences, compare notes on progress (Borsco et al., 1996), encourage each other and 'learn from each other's difficulties' (Cook, 1991). In other programmes such as 'The Edinburgh Listening Group', up to 10 CI recipients meet regularly to practise auditory training exercises, listening skills and speech production, and discuss telephone use and cochlear implant (CI) accessory management under the supervision of two therapists (A Kennedy, 2001, personal communication). Some programmes use different combinations of clinician pairs from their team of speech and language therapist, psychologist, phoniatrician and audiologist to run group training, because it is felt that it is necessary to provide different communication styles and avoid 'excessive involvement in the patient–client relationship' (Bosco et al., 1996). In the Montréal model, both the spouse or other support person *and* other CI recipients are included in structured psychosocial group-based learning programmes, described in more detail below. These 2-day workshops bring together five or six CI recipients, each with their support person (where applicable), for sharing and discussion of personal and practical aspects of living with a CI. Using a group problem-solving approach, the participants learn how to find solutions to frequently encountered communication problems (Hogan, 2001).

Do patients benefit from structured rehabilitation?

There is general agreement among those who practise in this area that patients vary in the degree to which they benefit from a programme of rehabilitation training. Edgerton (1985) described a number of factors that may affect the individual achievements of CI patients, including personality and motivation, pre-implant patient expectations, visual processing capabilities, family attitudes, the presence of other disabilities, auditory discrimination abilities with the CI and social–vocational history and status. In our experience these factors remain relevant. Other factors that may affect the effectiveness of a rehabilitation programme include problem-solving skills, attention span, metacommunication skills, and the degree of perseverance and completeness with which the patient undertakes the rehabilitation programme. The quality of the management offered and type of approach used by the therapist are also likely to affect outcome.

Certainly, much of the support for structured rehabilitation is anecdotal. Eisenberg and Berliner (1983) were among the first to document a post-implant training programme. Users of the single electrode implant were given training in building tolerance to sound, discrimination tasks to increase awareness and use of prosody in speech, voice monitoring practice and communication strategies. Music and environmental sounds were used in a multisensory approach to sound awareness training with prelingually deafened adults. The therapy programme was reported to make an important contribution to acclimatization to the implant. Cook (1991) describes a post-implant rehabilitation programme where the patient attends the clinic for two 3-day blocks one week apart, and then one day per month for up to a year. A highly organized home training programme using recorded material supports the training. The group observed that those who completed the course showed a steady improvement in perception and understanding of spoken language, whereas those who were unable to complete the formal training 'reached a virtual standstill' once the intervention ended.

Lansing and Davis (1988) looked at the effect of early versus delayed speech perception training for adult CI users. One group ($n = 5$) of CI recipients received intensive aural rehabilitation training at 1 month after switch-on whereas a second group ($n = 8$) did not receive any training until 9 months after switch-on. All CI recipients were tested immediately before and after training. Trends in the group mean data suggest that gains following early aural rehabilitation may exceed those achieved by implant use alone. In a follow-up study, Lansing and Davis (1990) reported on a group of 17 patients after 18 months and found that the advantage for the group receiving early training was maintained. Although the make-up of the groups has been questioned (Thompson, 1990), this study has provided some of the strongest evidence so far of the value of a systematic training programme in cochlear implantation.

Gagné et al. (1991) report the effectiveness of an intensive 12-week, individualized, post-implant rehabilitation programme for four patients. Speech perception tests were administered quarterly for a year. The results suggest that most of the improvement occurred soon after implantation. However, the authors were cautious about concluding that intensive auditory rehabilitation programmes are not effective. Informal enquiries revealed that participants reported benefit in the area of telephone communication and 'more effective use of communication strategies'. These two areas were not part of the formal evaluation. The evaluation also did not investigate changes in quality of life. Ceiling effects (i.e. where further improvement in performance would be very small because the patient is already achieving at a high level) in one subject may have confounded the results, and further improvements may have been shown for the subjects if testing in background noise had been part of the assessment. The study recommended an approach to audiological rehabilitation of CI recipients based on patient goals.

Gray et al. (1995) reported the results of an 18-month follow-up study of 15 postlingually deaf adult patients using the Ineraid implant after 10 hours of training and again at 9 and 18 months after implant. Much of the improvement in speech discrimination occurred after the initial 10 hours of intensive training with further improvement over the following 18 months. In elderly implant recipients, Watson et al. (2002) reported that attendance at one-on-one aural rehabilitation sessions positively affected speech perception outcomes.

Sherbourne et al. (2002) used self-report questionnaires to examine the effectiveness of a week-long intensive psychosocial rehabilitation programme for deafened adults (defined as 'an inability to use sound, aided or unaided, to follow speech') at the LINK Centre for Deafened People. The programme includes self-management, coping skills, confidence building, communication strategies and access to services. Statistically significant improvements after one month were demonstrated in psychological state, clinical depression, general health, quality of life, communication effectiveness and social functioning. The improvements were sustained over 6 months. This demonstrates just how powerful a client-focused programme, which addresses the needs of both the deafened person and the carer and focuses on the *adjustment* to hearing loss, can be, even without the technology of a cochlear implant.

It is important not to overlook the benefits reported by the patients from regular and structured rehabilitation. Feedback from those participating at our centre suggest that patients found the exercises provided some structure and direction in the first few weeks after switch-on, a time of many new experiences and feelings. Others reported that the exercises gave objective evidence that they were achieving and progressing. As Biderman (1998, pp. 35–6) writes in her account of her experience with an implant *Wired for Sound*: 'Rehabilitative work helped me to really see how much I could do and made me feel very good about what I could hear and understand . . . and the formal structured rehabilitation with a therapist reminded me repeatedly and irrefutably of my successes, large and small.' Some patients comment that the structured activities helped them to focus on hearing experiences after many years of being very visually oriented.

There are many questions that remain to be answered. These include what the most effective types of intervention are, what the optimal schedule for such a course is and which patients are most likely to benefit. Clinics are encouraged to adapt and evaluate the methods proposed below to suit their own needs.

Reducing the length of therapy

The financial implications of providing therapist time for a structured auditory and communication training programme have been a concern for some programmes. Four strategies are recommended to maximize efficiency: (1) initial screening of the patient's listening skills at entry into the programme, (2) a primary focus on key goals or areas of need identified *by the patient*, (3) home-based training and (4) use of a patient home manual or take-home material to supplement clinic training. These strategies are described in detail below.

The next section highlights the key features of what the authors have found to be an effective rehabilitation programme. Chapter 5 details a staged competency-based auditory training programme and its under-lying principles together with suggestions for communication therapy.

Recommended resource materials are presented. In Chapter 6, suggestions for forming a client-focused intervention plan are discussed.

Key features of the programme

Primary use of the auditory-alone modality

Objective

The objective is to maximize the use of the auditory component of the speech signal.

Rationale

Many patients presenting to an implant programme have been accustomed to a degraded auditory input and have learned to rely heavily on visual cues. Through dependence on the visual modality, many become good speech readers. However, their auditory skills are comparatively lacking. While acknowledging that audition-alone training is not representative of real-life communication (except for listening on the telephone), practice in a 'safe' environment can facilitate and enhance the decoding of auditory information. This is important because the CI recipient's new implant provides access to sounds (especially high frequencies) that may be unfamiliar and that the patient may not identify. Repeated audition-alone stimuli help encourage listening and help people to retrain and build confidence in the auditory sense. Unlike in real life, the CI user often feels comfortable enough in the clinical situation to make a guess, despite the risk of making errors and so *can receive focused and timely feedback*.

This enhancement of auditory decoding can facilitate the patient's use of combined audiovisual signals. In the CI user's own environment, of course, the use of speech reading will help the patient to integrate the new hearing sensations with the visual speech patterns and direct the listener's *attention* to speech rather than noise (for a summary of how visual information complements a degraded auditory signal see Summerfield, 1987).

The development of new speech-processing strategies over the past 15 years has led to significant increases in audition-alone, open-set, word-and-sentence discrimination. Wilson (2000) provides a comparative review of speech processing strategies and outcomes. Audition-alone, open-set sentence scores above 70% are now fairly common since the introduction of third generation cochlear implant speech processors, and new speech processing strategies (Parkinson et al., 2001; Dowell et al., 2002). These strategies include continuous interleaved sampling (CIS), spectral peak

(SPEAK) and advanced combination encoder (ACE). It would seem that, with the increased availability of auditory cues, the need for formal speech reading training in the implanted group is diminishing. However, Tye-Murray (1993) gives suggestions for designing a speech-reading training programme, if required.

Although the trend in outcomes from implantation is towards less dependency on visual cues, there will always be some individuals for whom the implant is primarily an aid to speech reading, particularly congenitally hearing-impaired adults. Modifying the exercises to provide visual cues for some, or all, of the stimulus will ensure that a balance is maintained between achievement and progress.

The programme begins at the patient's current level of functioning and ability

Objective

The objective is to increase time efficiency by commencing training at a level that is manageable, acknowledges current skill level and is sufficiently challenging for the patient.

Rationale

There is great variation in how much conversational speech will be understood in the first week after switch-on. It is important that the starting point for the auditory training reflects these differences. The following observations reflect the experience at our clinics. Patients who have been unaided or had no measurable hearing thresholds for many years may report that they can hear a variety of sounds when the therapist is speaking, but do not recognize any words or even patterns in words. Others will comment that they can immediately notice the difference between male and female voices, can recognize the rising inflexion of a question, and already hear differences in word length. CI recipients with severe-to-profound hearing loss preoperatively and/or those who demonstrated some aided benefit will often spontaneously comment that particular words or family names are distinguishable in a sentence. In CI users whose hearing loss is more recent or with a short period of profound deafness, it is not unusual for them to already recognize very familiar phrases such as 'Good morning' without visual cues.

Thus, some patients appear to have access to a high-fidelity auditory representation of speech very soon after switch-on and their rehabilitation programme may commence with more advanced skills such as telephone training and strategies for conversation in noise. Others appear from their performance to be using a more distorted representation of speech. The latter group presumably needs longer to extract the relevant information (Dorman et al., 1990). These CI recipients may commence with more analytical training and compensatory strategies. A speech perception screening assessment, such as that provided in the Nucleus 22 Channel Cochlear Implant System Rehabilitation Manual (Mecklenberg et al., 1986), can be used to establish the appropriate entry level for speech perception training. The importance of not allowing preliminary assessment of the CI recipients' skill levels to dominate the initial sessions cannot be over-emphasized. CI users who experience only assessment without therapy or the chance to achieve 'successes'/acquire some skills in the early sessions will quickly become discouraged and may abandon the rehabilitation programme (Erber, 1996, 2002).

Balancing the appropriate level of challenge with maintaining patient success

Objective

The objective is to train at a level that meets *and extends* the CI user's current abilities, while still allowing the CI recipient to be successful.

Rationale

The importance of building 'early successes' into a rehabilitation programme has been recognized for many years (e.g. Erber, 1982; Eisenberg, 1985). Compliance, motivation and morale are maintained when the patient is *achieving* in the programme. Speed of learning is increased when the CI user practises many similar items in a relatively short space of time, so-called 'drilling'. This focuses the CI user's attention on a particular feature and at the same time reinforces and consolidates the CI recipient's skills. However, it is important to include tasks that *extend* the CI recipient's abilities and exercise different skill areas to ensure optimum use of therapy time. As a broad guide, a success rate of 70% is sufficiently challenging to produce improvement with enough success to maintain motivation.

As CI recipients differ greatly in their speed of progress, the patient's skill level must be regularly reviewed so that the tasks remain challenging. Significant variation has been reported with respect to the timeframe in which gains are made in speech perception by CI recipients, e.g. some CI users make most gains in the first month, whereas others continue to show measured improvement up to several months or even several years after implant (Dorman et al., 1990; Spivak and Walzman, 1990; Tye-Murray et al.,

1992; Dorman and Loizou, 1997). Short- to medium-term gains may be related to gradual changes in the fidelity of the auditory representation of speech as a result of a more finely tuned speech processor. Dorman and Loizou (1997) cite central mechanisms of signal decoding as possible mechanisms to explain the longer-term gains.

Inclusion of frequent communication partners

Objective

The objective is to generalize skills learnt with the therapist to communication with people with whom the patient frequently interacts (frequent communication partner or FCP) and to other speakers.

Rationale

As the therapist steps into and out of the CI recipient's life for a relatively short time, the interaction with the therapist will be of limited value in the long term. The therapist's knowledge of conversational rules and strategies limits his or her use as a naïve conversational practice partner. A programme in which speech perception and compensatory skill training take place only in the clinic with the therapist is unlikely to result in generalization to the real world because it does not reproduce the many acoustically different voices, poor speaker habits that can degrade the speech signal, or the range of causes of communication breakdown.

The advantage of involvement of a FCP in post-implant rehabilitation is made overt to the CI recipient and his or her family early in the assessment process in our programmes. For those patients living alone, it is essential to work out before implantation who can take on the role of the regular conversation partner for the rehabilitation period. In our clinics we have found a number of sources successful. These include members of the immediate and extended family, neighbours, friends, work colleagues, nursing home personnel, church or religious associates, members of a patient's hobby group, local volunteer organizations, local hearing-impaired support group and other CI recipients living nearby.

Involving partners and/or the FCP in the auditory rehabilitation session can increase awareness of the limitations of the implant and methods to overcome these limitations. FCPs can learn how to use 'clear speech' (Picheny et al., 1985) as opposed to conversational speech, create good listening environments and adopt communication strategies that would better meet the patient's needs than those that were used before implantation. When conversation repair strategies are being explained, the support person can observe the therapist, especially *when* and *how* to intervene, and practise these interventions first in the clinic, then at home. There is much support for incorporating FCPs into the rehabilitation process (Eisenwort, 1985; Cooper, 1991; Tye-Murray, 1993; Erber, 2002; Lind, 2004).

Home practice and self-assessment

Objective

The objective is to generalize what has been practised in the clinic to other communication contexts, to expedite progress and to reduce clinic time.

Rationale

When home-based training is a key component of the intervention method, the therapist directs the training, and each auditory training exercise or strategy can be demonstrated and practised in the clinic, but a significant portion of *skill consolidation* can take place at home. Some 'drilling' occurs in the clinic to ensure that the task is appropriately challenging and that the patient understands the task and its purpose. Repetition of the task may continue until the patient begins to show the skill that is being practised. Ideally, the support person(s) should observe and then practise both the exercises and the appropriate method of assisting the CI recipient.

Home practice is encouraged on two levels: first, formal drill or 'focused practice' of a particular skill or feature – 15–30 minutes allows for practice of different tasks. In our experience CI recipients often spend longer on auditory tasks, suggesting that patient motivation, success and sense of achievement is high. Practising at the same time every day appears to make training an integral part of daily routine and increases compliance. Second, informal practice is encouraged, where the family provides increased incidental listening and interaction opportunities in the daily routine, such as commenting to the patient on what they are doing.

Home practice encourages the patient to generalize skills learned with the therapist to the environment in which patient communicates every day. The patient's own environment provides not only a variety of speakers, but also topics of relevance, greater realism (e.g. speakers are not always *focused* on talking directly to the CI recipient) and patient-specific environmental noise.

Use of a patient home manual (e.g. Wayner et al., 1998; Pedley, 2000; Plant, 2001) can reduce the time requirement in the clinic in a number of areas. Time spent on information counselling can be reduced by making available reference information on topics such as insurance, local support groups, basic troubleshooting and battery management, air travel and other frequently asked questions. This leaves more time available to address the patient's *specific* concerns and for rehabilitation. The home manual can provide written confirmation of the counselling and support given in the initial postoperative period (e.g. factors that can affect progress with the implant, experiences common to all CI recipients). This may facilitate and expedite understanding given the patient's initial speech perception skills post-implant. A home manual can provide a summary of communication tactics for the patient and the family to support the therapist's discussions and demonstrations. Inclusion of auditory training material saves time in sourcing and copying exercises for home use. However, it is important to provide instructions that detail exactly what is required, and make it clear to the patient and the conversation partner what skill is being practised. A troubleshooting section encourages and empowers the patient to problem solve, rather than calling the clinic. In some home training programmes the manual activities incorporate a report that is returned on a weekly basis to the clinician for assessment. The patient then receives feedback on progress in written form (Tye-Murray et al., 1996).

A daily diary or weekly report kept by the CI recipient can provide a valuable record of progress and can allow the therapist quickly to identify and focus on specific problems, areas of concern and issues of adjustment to the CI (Edgerton, 1985). For CI recipients with a long-standing hearing loss, regular journal entries may help the patient to focus on auditory experiences. The diary may suggest broad areas for entries or ask specific questions of both the CI recipient and the FCP (Tye-Murray et al., 1993).

For the CI user and family, a home manual for cochlear CI recipients provides a number of advantages:

• Awareness of his or her progress, building confidence and providing encouragement.
• A sense of empowerment for the individual: as well as the self-help suggestions in communication tactics and repair strategies, the daily listening journal can be used to record experiences in communication situations, any problems that arise, solutions that worked and how the patient might change his or her behaviour to solve a similar problem in the future (Robbins, 2000).
• Guidance notes on issues such as becoming accustomed to environmental sounds and listening to music through an implant, together with regular journal entries, remind the CI recipient to focus on auditory experiences.
• Specific feedback to family members about the limitations of the implant:

some family members notice for the first time the directionality of the speech processor microphone, or the CI recipient's difficulty with speech from a distance during home training.

- Direction and instructions for those family members who wish to help with the rehabilitation but cannot attend the clinic sessions.
- The convenience of ready access to training material or suggestions for suitable material at home. This is important when family members are working or have other dependants.
- A vehicle for documentation of issues to raise with the therapist, from either the CI recipient or those in close contact with him or her.

Individually tailored goals negotiated between CI recipient and therapist

Objective

The objective is to ensure that the training programme meets the CI user's expectations and needs.

Rationale

The programme focuses on the aims of the CI recipient. We have found this approach more effective and efficient than providing the same training with each CI recipient. Focusing on specific needs rather than aiming for general improvement in communication provides the CI recipient with feedback on progress in specific situations, making success easier to recognize (Wescott, 1994). By defining broad long-term goals at the outset of the programme (by discussing expectations and likely prognosis), the CI user and therapist can work together towards common goals rather than adopting competing or unrealistic goals. Examples of long-term goals are: to be able to talk with long-distance relatives by phone, to be able to converse confidently in group situations or to improve communication with work colleagues.

Table 4.1 shows an overview of the rehabilitation process. It can be seen that goals are continually refined during the course of rehabilitation. From the broad goals, the CI user and therapist identify specific goals. This will assist in planning the objectives for training in speech perception *and* compensatory skills because the two are interdependent. Once the auditory representation of speech through the implant becomes more finely tuned through mapping (see Chapter 3) and the therapist gains a better indication of the patient's ability to use the information, the goals can be adjusted to remain realistic and relevant.

Table 4.1 Staged approach to intervention

Stage	Practical aspects	Psychophysical aspects	Rehabilitation	Goals
Pre-implant	Demonstrate device	Audiological, medical and other assessments	Expectation counselling Programme outline Support counselling	Patient's preliminary goals
1. Switch-on	Processor management Equipment maintenance Precautions	Initial electrode activation Familiarize with mapping	Support counselling Begin listening practice for environmental sounds and own voice Assess speech perception ability Assess communication skills Address dynamics of family communication	Establish entry level of speech perception training Set broad goals
2. Refine map	ALD introduction Troubleshooting	Fine tune T and C levels Refine parameters Alternative processing strategies	Support counselling, i.e. identify specific listening problems Begin speech perception training Begin communication therapy Address dynamics of family relationships	Set specific goals

3. Stable map	ALDs in specific situations Independence in troubleshooting skills	Maintain map Go to stage 2 if indicated by continuing specific listening problems or poor progress Situation-specific maps	Support counselling i.e. identify specific listening problems and family issues Modify training to address above Advanced or specific communication skills training, e.g. groups, noise, phone, work Psychosocial workshop	Goals met or refined
4. Step down	Management of spares Procedure for obtaining loaner	Maintain map	Closure counselling Introduction to other support staff Support groups	Acknowledge goals achieved Acknowledge limitations Establish long-term goals
5. Maintenance	Supply spares Repairs	Maintain map Assess appropriateness of upgrades of processors and/or speech processing strategies and software features	Periodic assessment to review progress Coordinated support from non-clinical staff; CI recipient groups If change in situation, e.g. work, bereavement, go to stage 3	

ALDs, assistive listening devices.

In one example, a patient with good open-set discrimination in quiet has a broad goal of improving communication with work colleagues. Specific goals identified by the therapist and CI recipient include improving speech understanding in daily meetings in a noisy open-plan office, enhancing the acoustics of his or her immediate work area, increasing understanding about the limitations of the implant among work colleagues and improving the accuracy of understanding internal phone messages. In this case, training in several areas can be offered and these are discussed in Chapter 6.

In a second example, a CI recipient's broad goal might be to enjoy conversation with his or her own young children. The specific goals might be to enhance speech perception, particularly for *fast* speech, improve conversational skills, and improve or develop environmental tactics to assist in noisy environments such as the school (see Chapter 7). The therapist may adapt or modify auditory training exercises so that they are suitable for the CI recipient to practise with his or her children (in our experience, children enjoy role-playing QUEST?AR (Erber, 1996, 2002) with the hearing-impaired parent and auditory training activities using pictures). If the parent has a very longstanding hearing loss, one of the specific goals may be to demonstrate to the children how much the implanted parent can now hear or to teach the children about the implant itself. Another goal may be to help the CI recipient's partner to explore strategies for encouraging the children to go to the implanted parent when they need help.

Ownership of the goals is likely to increase commitment to, and interest in, the rehabilitation process, e.g. if telephone use is a CI user's stated broad goal, this can be incorporated into *each stage* of the auditory training rather than waiting for the CI recipient to achieve a certain level of open-set discrimination. Once a CI user discriminates family names from a closed set of names with ease, the same task can be practised by telephone. This extends the difficulty of the task (as the signal is heard through additional equipment which changes the sound quality), maintains relevance and targets the patient's goals. A CI user may state that his or her long-term goal is to retain a job that involves taking orders for machine parts over the telephone. By using the suggestions in Chapter 5 as a design guide, exercises using the part numbers can be created as a closed-set identification task, as an open-set recognition task and as a role-play with a single scripted conversation. Recognition of machine code numbers can be practised in quiet, in noise and then by telephone. In this way, the rehabilitation remains highly relevant to the patient's daily life.

The therapist must also pay attention to the goals when deciding on the length of time to offer formal training because some CI recipients will achieve their goals earlier than others.

As can be seen from Table 4.1, CI recipient goals may be redefined if the CI user experiences a major life change, such as death of a spouse, moving home or change of employment, e.g. a CI recipient who can no longer rely on the partner to assist with following a group conversation can be offered assistance to be more independent by practising compensatory strategies (such as use of situation and topic cues), practising clarification strategies and use of the lapel microphone, and may also be offered assertiveness training.

Therapist flexibility to maintain CI user cooperation

Objective

The objective is to ensure that therapy is stimulating, relevant and challenging for the CI recipient.

Rationale

A flexible approach to both the level and content of training material is important. The therapist may need to alter the level of difficulty of an exercise 'on-line' (i.e. during the session) to reflect the patient's changing abilities.

To maintain the CI user's interest, increase relevance and incorporate a variety of styles of information presentation (e.g. prose, notes, dialogue, descriptive and technical), a clinic should aim to collect and use a variety of materials. Examples are special interest magazines (e.g. gardening, cooking, travel), graded reader novels, local newspapers, testimonials written by CI recipients, recipes, local maps and a children's encyclopaedia. CI recipients can be encouraged to bring in their own periodicals, work-related material or special interest books. Attention should be paid to the individual's literacy level, particularly with those who were born with some degree of hearing loss and those for whom English is a second language. The approach to rehabilitation may also need to be modified to take account of the individual's cultural needs. A comprehensive list of auditory training and communication therapy resources is given in Chapter 5.

Frequently changing tasks is a characteristic of the therapist's adaptable approach to the programme. This ensures that the patient does not become fatigued or bored with a particular activity. As an example, a session may include a 3-minute segment of tracking task (see Chapter 5, exercise 3k), a brief period of audiovisual work, audition-alone synthetic tasks working on a specific compensatory strategy, an interactive instruction following task with the spouse working with the patient so that the therapist can observe repair strategies, an exercise in noise using a specific assistive listening device (see Chapter 11) and a short telephone exercise.

It is a good idea to use a number of different learning modalities because not all adults learn in the same way, e.g. a programme could incorporate a combination of written stimuli, visual tasks or stimuli, spoken presentation, recorded material, computer-based learning and audiovisual presentation. As many programmes do not have the resources to provide complex technical support, the rehabilitation programme described in Chapter 5 is designed to be directed by an experienced therapist, to use the CI recipient's own support network together with a take-home manual or material.

It is important for the therapist not to pre-judge the likely outcome of rehabilitation for a CI user, because performance can too easily be limited by expectations that are set too low and become a self-fulfilling prophecy. Cases where a CI recipient's internal device has been compromised in some way, or where the patient has experienced many years of no auditory input, might erroneously lead the therapist to expect poorer outcomes. In addition, progress in the first month should not be taken as a guide to long-term outcomes. Dorman et al. (1990) report that some CI users who achieved very poor word recognition score at one month post-implant went on to produce above-average scores 1–2 years after implant.

Training generalized more easily into daily living by incorporating activities requiring two-way interaction

Objective

The objective is to ensure that therapy is transferred into everyday situations.

Rationale

Activities that engage the CI recipient and the practice partner in true two-way interaction provide an important progression from 'listen–respond' tasks. Conversation-like activities afford the clinician an opportunity to observe the CI recipient and the FCP in a more conversationally realistic situation, and to adopt a problem-solving approach to those elements of the interaction that reduce conversational fluency and build skills that can be transferred into daily life. Examples of interactive exercises are those that involve the exchange of information to complete a task and role-playing. Interactive activities allow aspects of communication therapy such as conversational partner management (see Chapter 7) to be integrated into the rehabilitation sessions. This type of activity can be used as a vehicle to increase participation, confidence and assertiveness of the patient. In our experience, many CI recipients and their families report a marked reduction in conversation in the period before implantation as a result of the difficulties imposed by the hearing loss. In some cases this period may be several years. In such cases, re-training in conversational skills is an essential component of the rehabilitation process. Interactive exercises can also be structured into increasing levels of difficulty to extend the patient's skills progressively.

Incidental practice and training in conversation control and strategies to repair conversational breakdown

Objective

The objective is to provide opportunities for the patient to practise initiating conversation 'repairs' in a 'safe' environment with a familiar speaker. The aim of this process is to increase patient independence in managing communication misunderstandings.

Rationale

Many CI recipients have limited awareness of the *range* of repair strategies and may benefit from the opportunity to practise those with which the CI recipient is less familiar (Tye-Murray, 1991; Tye-Murray et al., 1993). In *all stages* of the programme, the therapist attempts to reduce the patient's reliance on the therapist to resolve instances of conversation breakdown. By gradually reducing the amount of spontaneous assistance given, the CI recipient is forced to use repair strategies such as asking for a segment to be repeated or rephrased, or use limited-choice questions (see Chapter 6) when they have not heard or only partially understood. The therapist provides positive reinforcement when the CI recipient spontaneously uses a repair strategy, but this is gradually withdrawn as the therapist comes to expect the CI user to initiate repair more frequently. By practising with the therapist, the CI recipient may become increasingly assertive and willing to generalize the skill to FCPs and in more challenging communicative contexts, such as outside the home. Incorporating communication repair into the rehabilitation programme is supported by a number of authors (Cooper, 1991; Tye-Murray, 1991).

Adoption of holistic approach

Objective

The objective is to consider other needs of the CI recipient apart from their immediate auditory rehabilitation needs.

Rationale

In our experience, a CI user is more likely to progress and attend to training if his or her other needs are addressed, concurrently where possible. These include:

- Psychological needs such as issues of self-esteem, fear of failure, relationship counselling.
- Medical needs may have to be considered in relation to issues such as appointment scheduling (e.g. a CI recipient may be taking medication at certain times of day that may affect concentration and attention span, or a CI recipient may be unable to sit for long periods because of circulatory problems).
- Physical needs, such as a blind person needing training material in advance to translate into Braille, or device management for a CI recipient with severe arthritis.
- Specific environmental needs: the CI recipient's working and/or social environment should be discussed in detail so that potential problems and difficulties can be addressed *before* the issue becomes problematic. This may include wet, humid or dusty environments, or the specific noise of the CI recipient's workplace or classroom, e.g. for a CI recipient who began working in a restaurant kitchen, special attention was given to methods of keeping moisture out of the speech processor.

A holistic approach can also be applied to each training goal, e.g. when teaching telephone use, the therapist may consider ergonomics, convenience, cost issues, technical issues such as choice of telecoil, phone adapter or speaker phone (see Chapter 11) as well as which telephone strategy best suits the CI user's abilities (e.g. telephone code, closed-set telephone message list or open-set phone use). Telephone strategies are covered in Chapters 7 and 10.

Addition of other factors to increase the difficulty of tasks

Objective

The objective is to address CI user-reported difficulties in specific, real-life communication settings and to extend the skill level of CI recipients who are coping well in ideal conditions.

Rationale

The performance of the CI recipient in the almost ideal situation provided by the clinic (quiet room, familiar, trained and focused speaker) is unlikely to provide a representative sample of the CI recipient's real-life abilities. It is therefore important that the *reported difficulties* in other communicative contexts be taken into account when providing auditory training. There are a number of situations that can be recreated in the clinic for training purposes.

Difficulty hearing in background noise can be simulated using multi-talker babble beginning at high signal-to-noise ratios (SNRs) (e.g.+ 20 dB SNR), a recorded narrative or a radio (music and talkback shows provide different challenges). Sometimes, the CI user may report difficulty managing in a specific background sound such as an air-conditioning fan or distant factory floor noise. Some CI recipients may be willing to make a recording of the noise so that multiple solutions may be tested in the clinic such as mapping changes, optimizing use of speech processor controls, assistive listening devices (see Chapter 11) and/or learning to make more effective use of compensatory cues.

Practice listening to unfamiliar speakers can be achieved through the involvement of family members (see above) or other clinic staff, and use of recorded books or TV programmes. For difficulty following fast speech, which is common in elderly CI recipients, training can be given in processing progressively accelerated samples of speech. For difficulty with auditory memory, training can be provided with progressively longer sentences to practise strategies such as listening for key words.

Difficulty interpreting degraded speech signals may occur with heavily accented speech or when the speaker turns the head away. The CI user can practise auditory tasks with recorded speech of different accents, and with the speaker in different positions (facing, speech from behind and with the therapist moving around the room). The effectiveness of contextual cues and prediction to assist with auditory closure can be demonstrated.

Regular assessments

Objective

The objective is to determine and document changes in the CI recipient's performance and assess outcomes of implantation.

Rationale

Repeated assessments are employed to monitor improvements in each patient's performance and indicate the efficacy of the rehabilitation programme. An evaluation of function of the internal device should precede formal testing where possible. If recent adjustment to a patient's MAP has caused significant changes in sound perception, it may be more appropriate to defer the assessment until the patient has had time to adjust to the new settings. Assessments may evaluate speech perception with and without lip-reading, changes in speech production, communication skills, recognition of environmental sounds and quality-of-life measures.

The combined information from assessments can be used to:

- demonstrate progress in speech perception ability and view these improvements in light of responses to quality-of-life measures
- obtain information to develop new auditory and communication training objectives
- consider whether modifications to device programming are necessary
- assess the extent to which preoperative expectations and objectives have been met; this information can be particularly useful to counsel the patient in the closure phase (e.g. to modify patient expectations where applicable)
- ensure that performance has not decreased, because this may indicate problems requiring further investigation.

For audiological measures, a test battery approach (i.e. use of a number of different measures) is necessary to probe different levels of speech perception and cater for a range of performance of CI recipients. The test battery should include words both in isolation and in the context of sentences. Discrimination errors on single word tasks can indicate that certain acoustic cues are either not available to, or not being used by, the CI user. Sentence testing may also demonstrate the extent to which a patient uses context, semantics and prediction. Consonant/vowel confusion testing, such as that originally described by Miller and Nicely (1955), can be used to indicate which acoustic features of speech are 'used' and which are confused, and therefore require further training. This information may, in turn, shed light on the difficulties described by the patient.

In our experience, the performance levels of postlingually deafened CI recipients are now such that the most useful speech material is open set sentences and words. Partly this is attributable to the development of better speech processing strategies and partly it results from the criteria for implantation having changed such that some CI recipients already have some open-set discrimination ability pre-implantation, albeit limited. Recordings of sentence tests in noise are increasingly necessary to be able to show continued improvements in speech perception after implantation, i.e. to avoid ceiling effects. For a more detailed discussion of the issues to be considered in developing a test battery, see Dowell et al. (1990).

Repeated assessments performed with and without lip-reading can provide an indication of the patient's increasing ability to integrate the auditory and visual information. These assessments can be performed live voice or, better still, using a video-recorded speech test. When possible, the recorded speech should be in the same accent as the patient's. Measures of speech perception with visual cues are particularly important in providing encouragement to patients whose open-set audition-alone speech perception scores remain low. Such patients may show significant improvements in audition plus vision scores, compared with the pre-implant scores in the same condition. In some patients, combining auditory and visual information works to significant advantage: the scores for audition plus vision condition are greater than addition of the auditory-alone and vision-alone scores. This phenomenon is referred to as superadditivity (Dorman, 1993).

Audiological measures should not be used in isolation, because they provide information only about the patient performance in speech recognition in the clinic, in an artificial test situation. This is usually in a quiet or sound-treated room, with none of the environmental factors present that can degrade the intended message. As discussed in the assessment of communication needs (see Chapter 2), baseline measures of a CI recipient's communication profile and QoL self-assessment specific to hearing disability (e.g. Hawthorne et al., 2004) may provide information about his or her functional communication ability and form an important part of assessing the outcome of implantation. Other measures that could be considered are the Glasgow Benefit Inventory (GBI) (Robinson et al., 1996) which measures hearing participation, focusing on independence levels, personal and social relationships, and adjustment to deafness. Also the Communication Profile for the Hearing Impaired (CPHI) (Demorest and Erdman, 1987) has been a useful assessment tool for communication skills including communication strategies, communication effectiveness at home and work, and personal adjustment such as acceptance of loss and withdrawal. Questionnaires designed for specific CI user groups have been reported. Horn et al. (1991) constructed a questionnaire for elderly implant recipients that explored areas such as ease of operation, extent of device use and functional benefits such as voice monitoring, confidence and participation in social activities.

If measures such as DYALOG (Erber, 1998, 2002) were used preoperatively to evaluate conversational performance, then ongoing assessments should be undertaken at key milestones postoperatively in order to monitor progress in this dimension.

CI recipients may score well in speech perception tests but their answers to QoL questions may indicate an inability to transfer these skills to the real world. Such discrepancies can direct the therapist to explore the patient's further needs, such as specific communication strategies, assertiveness training, a need for support with assistive listening devices (see Chapter 9) or participation in a psychosocial workshop (see Hogan, 2001). Conversely, patients may not perform well on speech perception tests but pre- and postoperative comparisons of QoL questions may show significant improvement. This can be an important counselling tool.

Tye-Murray et al. (1992) reported that environmental sound recognition improved gradually, up to 18 months after switch-on. In our experience, CI recipients are now recognizing environmental sounds soon after switch-on. This could be caused by the increased frequency content of information now provided by enhanced speech processing strategies. This skill is also affected by the context in which the sounds are heard. In our clinic, CI users self-evaluate environmental sound recognition by checking off an environmental sounds list (based on the 'Listening Check List' originally compiled by Plant, 1984) once the patient has learned to recognize each sound without visual cues. In our experience this is achieved comprehensively and quickly in the first month. For this reason we no longer perform periodic assessments of environmental sound recognition. However, the Iowa Environmental Sounds Test can be used if desired.

Improvements in speech and language can be formally assessed before and after implantation and rehabilitation. The changes that occur in speech production as a result of postlingual deafness may include inappropriate use of stress and pitch patterns, loudness levels, errors of articulation and aberrations in voice quality. As many adults do not show significant improvements in speech production apart from decreased voice *loudness*, many clinics may feel that it is not worth assessing this aspect.

This may change, however, with the new generation of cochlear implants and speech processors. Some authors have reported significant improvements in speech production, e.g. Dawson et al. (1995) reported that half of a group of participants aged over 8 years showed significant improvements over time on a test of articulation postoperatively compared with preoperative scores. One of two prelinguistically deafened adults in the study significantly improved on the articulation test. In our programme we have observed changes in speech and language abilities in some cases. These have included improvements in voice quality, a decrease in some speech production errors and an increase in new vocabulary usage, e.g. a young woman who was born with a moderate hearing loss was implanted in her mid-20s by which time she had been profoundly deaf for three years. After implant she acquired an ability to use the appropriate morphological markers to mark tense, e.g. 'ed' or 't'. Her family also remarked that she began to use many new colloquial phrases and expressions during the first year after implant.

In deciding when and how frequently to perform assessments, the clinician should be mindful of a number of issues: first, the time period in which stabilization of performance occurs. Patients appear to differ widely in their rate of accommodation to the hearing sensations produced by electrical stimulation. Some patients have high open-set scores immediately after switch-on. Tye-Murray et al. (1992) reported that performance improved up to 18 months but further improvements from 18 to 30 months may be small. Second, there is individual variation not only in the time course over which improvements in performance occur (Dorman et al., 1990), but also in which skills improve (Tye-Murray et al., 1992). Changes in performance over time may also be related to which device was implanted (Weston and Waltzman, 1995). Hence it may be useful to obtain measures preoperatively, at switch-on and at several intervals in the first 18 months. As mentioned above, one of the purposes of assessment is early detection of problems. Therefore, we recommend continued assessment on an annual basis.

Caution is needed in comparing performance after the same time period after implant across patients, because time and *experience* are not necessarily equivocal. Experience with the implant depends on the number of hours that the processor is worn and opportunities for interaction since 'switch-on'.

Attendance at a 1- or 2-day workshop addressing psychosocial issues associated with deafness and implantation

Objective

The objective is to heighten awareness of the emotional and psychological impact of hearing loss, and to enhance the capacity to manage day-to-day communication difficulties.

Rationale

Many of the activities offered to CI recipients in the clinic do not reproduce the psychosocial difficulties of managing potentially stigmatizing social situations and interpersonal dynamics. The exercises offered within the workshop provide participants with the opportunity to develop competencies in managing more demanding and complex communication situations.

The workshop offers a group-sharing and problem-solving approach, and ranges over several areas, some of which may be omitted depending on the ages and needs of the patients. In our programmes, the workshop is offered to the CI recipient and the FCP at around three months after implant when a stable representation of speech has been obtained, and the CI user and FCP more fully appreciate the limitations of the device and are therefore more motivated to find solutions to communication difficulties that remain. The areas are:

- The CI user recognizing the impact of the hearing loss on him- or herself and those around the patient
- Communication styles, e.g. assertiveness
- Communication as a source of stress and stress management
- Managing difficult communication environments, e.g. planning, environmental strategies
- Exploring the effects of hearing loss on relationship formation and maintenance
- Awareness of dependency issues, e.g. helpful and unhelpful caring
- Discussion of role changes
- Communication issues in the workplace
- Assistive listening devices.

The use of group work as a component of rehabilitation is supported by a number of authors (Cooper, 1991; Gagné et al., 1991). CI user reports suggest that confidence, assertiveness and self-esteem appear to improve after the course. Some CI recipients also report a reduction in anxiety associated with communication situations. Binzer (2002) used pre- and post-CPHI self-report assessment to evaluate the benefits of a 2-day psychosocial workshop. Changes on the personal adjustment scale (e.g. self-acceptance, anger, acceptance of hearing loss) were reported. A quarter of respondents showed an improvement on the self-acceptance scale. Over half of partners thought that the CI users were using more verbal strategies after the workshop. The DYALOG method (Erber, 1998) for measuring the time spent in conversational breakdown in a 10-minute segment of videotaped conversation was also used. The time spent in breakdown reduced significantly after the workshop and CI users were noted to make more use of specific rather than general conversation repair strategies.

Variation in service delivery for specific populations

Objective

The objective is to ensure that service provision meets each CI recipient's needs.

Rationale

Rehabilitation and training programmes may need to be modified to meet the needs of out-of-town CI user or individuals with special needs. An example of an appointment schedule for a local CI recipient may be: initially attending the clinic for two or three sessions of 2–3 hours for the initial switch-on, followed by weekly sessions for 1–2 months, monthly sessions for up to the first 3–4 months, and then 3-monthly sessions until the end of the first year. The patient may be seen once or twice a year thereafter.

Consider an out-of-town CI recipient, or one who may find it difficult to take time off work. In this case it may be more convenient, but just as effective, to see the CI user for two to three full days during the first week and then to bring the patient back for two to three consecutive days of training at 1 month after switch-on rather than weekly. The patient then reverts to a monthly to 3-monthly pattern as progress allows. In the case of students, switch-on and initial intensive rehabilitation may take place over 2–3 weeks during a vacation, with follow-up and further mapping and rehabilitation support between semesters.

CI recipients who demonstrate additional difficulties, such as auditory processing problems, may benefit from more frequent and intensive training with the therapist.

Acknowledgements

The objectives of Chapter 4 are based on the programmes offered at two cochlear implant centres: the New Zealand Cochlear Implant Programme in Auckland, NZ and the Queensland Cochlear Implant Centre in Brisbane, Australia. The authors would also like to acknowledge the input from colleagues and experience gained at the Manchester CI Programme, the Regional Audiology Unit at Withington Hospital, Manchester and the Hear and Say Centre, Brisbane, which have contributed to the philosophies and ideas expressed in this chapter. The works of Nancy Tye-Murray, Norm Erber and Geoff Plant have played important roles in the direction that our programmes have taken and the activities used. Carolina Puleston is acknowledged for kindly undertaking the documentation of the New Zealand CI programme in 2000, which formed the basis for Chapters 4 and 5. The objectives presented there have been found to be useful, manageable and acceptable to patients, as well as being effective in developing speech perception and communication skills.

References

Biderman B (1998) Wired for Sound: A journey into hearing. Toronto: Trifolium Books Inc.
Binzer SM (2002) Washington University adult aural rehabilitation programme – development and results. Presented at Cochlear Ltd Adult Psychosocial Seminar. September 2002, Manchester

Borsco E, Ballantyne D, Argiro MT (1996) Rehabilitation procedures adapted to adults and children. In: Allum DJ (ed.), Cochlear Implant Rehabilitation in Children and Adults. London: Whurr, 180–98

Cook BO (1991) Testing and rehabilitation of cochlear implant patients at the department of Audiology, Ssonderjukhuset, Stockholm. In: Cooper H (ed.), Cochlear Implants: A practical guide. London: Whurr Publishers, 240–50

Cooper H (1991) Training and rehabilitation for cochlear implant users. In: Cooper H (ed.), Cochlear Implants: A practical guide. London: Whurr Publishers, 219–39

Dawson PW, Blamey PJ, Dettman LC et al. (1995) A clinical report on speech production of cochlear implant users. Ear and Hearing 16: 551–61

Demorest ME, Erdman SA (1987) Development of the communication profile for the hearing impaired. Journal of Speech and Hearing Disorders 52: 129–43

Dorman MF (1993) Speech perception by adults. In: Tyler RS (ed.), Cochlear Implants: Audiological foundations. San Diego, CA: Singular Publishing Group, 145–90

Dorman MF, Loizou PC (1997) Changes in speech intelligibility as a function of time and signal processing strategy for an Ineraid patient fitted with continuous interleaved sampling (CIS) processors. Ear and Hearing 18: 147–55

Dorman MF, Dankowski K, McCandless G, Parkin JL, Smith L (1990) Longitudinal changes in word recognition by patients who use the Ineraid cochlear implant. Ear and Hearing 11: 455–9

Dowell RC, Brown AM, Mecklenburg DF (1990) Clinical assessment of implanted deaf adults. In: Clark GM, Tong YC, Patrick JF (eds), Cochlear Prostheses. Edinburgh: Churchill Livingstone, 193–205

Dowell RC, Hollow R, Winton E, Krauze K, Winfield E (2002). Outcomes for adults using cochlear implants: rethinking selection criteria. Paper presented at the Seventh International Cochlear Implant Conference, Manchester, UK, 4-6 September 2002.

Edgerton B (1985) Rehabilitation and training of postlingually deaf adult cochlear implant patients. Seminars in Hearing 6: 65–88

Eisenberg LS (1985) Training strategies for the post-implant patient. In: Schindler RA. Merzenich MM (eds), Cochlear Implants. New York: Raven Press, 511–15

Eisenberg LS, Berliner K I (1983) Rehabilitative procedures for the cochlear implant patient. Journal of the Academy of Rehabilitative Audiology 16: 104–13

Eisenwort B (1985) Rehabilitation of the post-implant patient. In: Schindler RA, Merzenich MM (eds), Cochlear Implants. New York: Raven Press, 517–520

Eisenwort B, Baumgartner W, Willinger U, Gstottner W, Frank F (1996) Maximising overall communication abilities for adult cochlear implant and hearing aid users. In: Allum DJ (ed.), Cochlear Implant Rehabilitation in Children and Adults. London: Whurr, 243–53

Erber NP (1982) Auditory Training. Washington DC: A.G. Bell Association for the Deaf.

Erber NP (1988) Communication Therapy for Hearing Impaired Adults. Abbotsford: Clavis

Erber NP (1996) Communication Therapy for Adults with Sensory Loss, 2nd edn. Melbourne: Clavis

Erber NP (1998) DYALOG: a computer-based performance measure of conversational performance. Journal of the Academy of Rehabilitative Audiology 31: 69–76

Erber NP (2002) Hearing, Vision, Communication, and Older People. Melbourne: Clavis

Gagné J, Parnes LS, LaRocque M, Hassan R, Vidas S (1991) Effectiveness of an intensive speech perception training program for adult cochlear implant recipients. Annals of Otology, Rhinology and Laryngology 100: 700–7

Gray RF , Quinn SJ, Court I, Vanat Z, Baguley DM (1995) Patient performance over eighteen months with the Ineraid intracochlear implant. Annals of Otology, Rhinology and Laryngology 166(suppl): 275–7

Hawthorne G, Hogan A, Giles E, Stewart M, Kethel L, White K, Plaith B, Pedley K, Rushbrooke E, Taylor A (2004) Evaluating the health-related quality of life effects of cochlear implants: a prospective study of an adult cochlear implant program. International Journal of Audiology 43: 183-192.

Hogan A (2001) Hearing Rehabilitation for Deafened Adults – A psycho-social approach. London: Whurr Publishers

Horn KL, McMahon NB, McMahon DC, Lewis JS, Barker M, Gherini S (1991) Functional use of the Nucleus 22-channel cochlear implant in the elderly. Laryngoscope 101: 284-8

Hull RH (1976) A linguistic approach to the teaching of speech – reading: theoretical and practical concepts. Journal of the Academy of Rehabilitative Audiology 9: 14-19

Jeffers J, Barley M (1971) Speechreading (Lipreading). Springfield, IL: Charles C Thomas

Kaplan G, Bally S J, Garretson C (1995) Speechreading – a way to improve understanding. Washington DC: Clerc Books

Lansing CR, Davis JM (1988) Early versus delayed speech perception training for adult cochlear implant users: initial results. Journal of Academy of Rehabilitative Audiology 21: 29-41

Lansing CR, Davis JM (1990) Evaluating the relative contribution of aural rehabilitation and experience to communication performance of adult cochlear implant users: preliminary data. In: Olswang LB, Thompson CK, Warren LS (eds), Treatment Efficacy Research in Communication Disorders. Rockville, MD: American Speech Language and Hearing Foundation, pp. 215-21

Lind C (2004) Conversation therapy following cochlear implantation. In: Pedley K, Lind C, Hunt P (eds), Adult Aural Rehabilitation – A guide for CI professionals. Sydney: Cochlear Ltd, in press

Mecklenberg DJ, Dowell RC, Jenison VW (1986) Nucleus 22 Channel Cochlear Implant System Rehabilitation Manual. Sydney: Cochlear Ltd

Miller GA, Nicely PE (1955) An analysis of perceptual confusions among some English consonants. Journal of the Acoustical Society of America 27: 338-52

Parkinson AJ, Arcaroli J, Staller SJ, Arndt PL, Cosgriff MD, Ebinger K (2001) The Nucleus 24 Contour cochlear implant system: adult clinical trial results. Poster presented at The American Academy of Audiology, San Diego, CA.

Pedley K (2000) Summary of the main features of the Queensland Cochlear Implant Centre Rehabilitation Program. Paper presented to the Australian Cochlear Implant Interest Group Inaugural Annual Conference, Adelaide, May 2000

Picheny MA, Durlach NI, Braida LD (1985) Speaking clearly for the hard of hearing I: intelligibility differences between clear and conversational speech. Journal of Speech and Hearing Research 28: 96-103

Plant G (1984) COMMTRAM. A Communication Training Program for Profoundly Deaf Adults. Sydney: National Acoustics Laboratories

Plant G (2001) Auditrain. Innsbruck, Austria: MED-EL

Robbins AM (2000) Rehabilitation after cochlear implantation. In: Niparko JK (ed.), Cochlear Implants: Principles and practices. Philadelphia, PA: Lippincott Williams & Wilkins, pp. 323-63

Robinson K, Gatehouse S, Browning GG (1996) Measuring patient benefit from otorhinolaryngological surgery and therapy. Annals of Otorhinolaryngology 105: 415-22

Sherbourne K, White L, Fortnuni H (2002) Intensive rehabilitation programmes for deafened men and women: an evaluation study. International Journal of Audiology 41: 195-201

Spivak LG, Waltzman SB (1990) Performance of cochlear implant patients as a function of time. Journal of Speech and Hearing Research 33: 511-19

Strauss-Schier A, Rost U (1996) Rehabilitation in adult cochlear implant patients. In: Allum D J (ed.), Cochlear Implant Rehabilitation in Children and Adults. London: Whurr, 254–65

Summerfield AQ (1987) Lip-reading and speech perception: Theoretical perspectives. In: B Dodd, R Campbell (eds), Hearing by Eye: The psychology of lip-reading. London: Lawrence Erlbaum, 3–52.

Thompson CK (1990) Issues in treatment efficacy research: comments on Doyle et al., Bourgeois, and Lansing and Davis papers. In: Olswang LB, Thompson CK, Warren LS (eds), Treatment Efficacy Research in Communication Disorders. Rockville: American Speech Language and Hearing Foundation, 223–231

Tye-Murray N (1991) Repair strategy usage by hearing-impaired adults and changes following communication therapy. Journal of Speech and Hearing Research 34: 921–8

Tye-Murray N (1993) Aural rehabilitation and patient management. In: Tyler RS (ed.), Cochlear Implants: Audiological foundations. San Diego, CA: Singular Publishing Group, 87–145

Tye-Murray N, Witt S (1997) Communication strategies training. Seminars in Hearing 18: 153–65

Tye-Murray N, Tyler RS, Woodworth GG, Gantz BJ (1992) Performance over time with a Nucleus or Ineraid cochlear implant. Ear and Hearing 13: 200–9

Tye-Murray N, Knutson JF, Lemke JH (1993) Assessment of communication strategies use: questionnaires and daily diaries. Seminars in Hearing 14: 388–51

Tye-Murray N, Spencer L, Witt S, Gilbert Bedia E (1996) Parent- and patient- centred aural rehabilitation. In Allum DJ (ed.), Cochlear Implant Rehabilitation in Children and Adults. London: Whurr, 65–82

Watson SD, Comer LK, Reilley D, Backous DD (2002) Cochlear implants in patients greater than 80 years of age. Poster presented at the 7th International Cochlear Implant Conference, September 2002, Manchester, UK

Wayner DS, Abrahamson JE, Casterton J (1998) Learning to Hear Again with a Cochlear Implant. Hear Again, Inc., 1200 Madison Ave, Austin, TX, USA

Westcott S (1994) Designing a communication training program for adults with acquired profound hearing loss. Paper presented at Advanced issues in Paediatric services, hearing aid fitting and hearing rehabilitation. Seminar–Workshop, NAL Sydney, October 1994.

Weston SC, Waltzman SB (1995) Performance as a function of time: a study of three cochlear implant devices. Annals of Otology, Rhinology and Laryngology 104(suppl 165): 19–24

Wilson B (2000) Strategies for representing speech information with cochlear implants. In: Niparko JK (ed.), Cochlear Implants: Principles and practices. Philadelphia, PA: Lippincott Williams & Wilkins, 129–69

Chapter 5
Aural rehabilitation following cochlear implantation: a staged approach to auditory training

KAREN PEDLEY AND ELLEN GILES

This chapter aims to provide the rehabilitationist with suggested materials for a heirarchical training guide of structured listening exercises. The materials and methods used in this programme use the following underlying principles.

Skills acquired in a hierarchical manner

Most practitioners agree that auditory training for people with a cochlear implant is best arranged in a hierarchical fashion. This is based on the CI recipient's progress in his or her development of listening skills, from one stage to the next (see, for example, Erber, 1982, 1996, 2002). Pre-testing identifies at which level in this sequence the CI user functions. Goals and training are then established to enable the CI recipient to progress to the next level. The hierarchy is reflected in the type of task and the complexity of the material used to accomplish a goal.

The exact nomenclature varies somewhat between authors. Tye-Murray (1993) describes examples of four levels of tasks: awareness, discrimination, identification and comprehension. Cooper (1991) describes five stages of speech perception training:

1. Detection: awareness of the presence or absence of sounds and gross speech features.
2. Discrimination: awareness of differences between two sounds where the patient indicates only whether the stimuli are the same or different. The

105

target difference may be: words of same or different syllable number; two monosyllabic words with the same or different vowel such as 'hid' and 'had'; sentence length; or a phrase read with the same or different intonation (e.g. rising or falling).

3. Identification: selecting a particular response from a 'closed-set' or finite list of possibilities. An identification task can be: selecting one word from a set where each has a different number of syllables; a set of different words that are related by topic; a set of words that differ only by the initial consonant; or identifying a sentence from a set of different or similar length sentences.

4. Recognition: identifying a sound, possibly with clues but without a set of possibilities, i.e. 'open-set' task. In this task the patient identifies the stimuli or sound spoken. The assumption here is that the patient can repeat the sound without understanding it.

5. Comprehension: attach meaning to the sound that he or she has identified. This task would demonstrate that the patient understands what is said. Examples of such tasks include answering questions about him- or herself, making up a question to an answer, following an instruction, or listening to a short passage and answering related questions.

In the programme described in this book, auditory training material is arranged into three stages: discrimination, identification and recognition/ comprehension.

From our clinical experience, the number of cochlear implant (CI) recipients who are unable to detect and discriminate sounds is very small (2–3%). Therefore the detection stage in training is targeted in only a small component of the session, e.g. detecting a small set of vowel and consonant sounds after each MAP (see Chapter 3) before the start of auditory training. Therefore detection is not discussed further. The number of activities at the discrimination level is also comparatively small because many CI recipients quickly demonstrate an ability to perceive whether the stimuli are the same or different, presumably as a result of excellent temporal pattern resolution and an ability to perceive intensity variations. In fact, in our experience, many postlingually deafened adults with implants who use third-generation speech-processing strategies demonstrate recognition skills soon after implantation. A number of researchers have also reported word recognition soon after implantation (Dorman, 1993; Parkinson et al., 2001). For this reason, most of the auditory training suggestions are at the identification and recognition/ comprehension levels.

Cooper's final two stages, recognition and comprehension, are combined into one stage in this programme – level three – because we believe that, to some degree, recognition relies on the ability to comprehend, whether deliberately or subconsciously. This is particularly true as task complexity and sentence length increase, so that the patient relies more on auditory memory and contextual cues, when available.

Optimal training programme including different levels of speech stimuli

Activities in attending to individual features or components of speech can be used alongside activities that require the patient to listen to whole phrases or sentences in a complementary manner.

Tye-Murray (1993) classifies training activities into two levels – phonetic and phrase/sentence level – and states that training at both levels is preferable. Phonetic-level tasks emphasize phonemic contrasts such as the voiced consonant (v) and unvoiced consonant (f) in the words *vale* and *fail.* Phrase- and sentence-level material could be the same words *fail* and *vale* but with a carrier sentence.

Cooper (1991) describes training material as analytical or synthetic (see Cooper, 1991, Figure 14.1, p. 226). In analytical training the focus is on:

- suprasegmental cues such as syllable number, intonation and stress
- segmental cues such as listening to nonsense syllables with contrasting pairs of consonants (e.g. aba, aka), or vowel pairs presented in isolation or in words in which the vowel is initially prolonged and then spoken with natural duration, e.g. *sheep* vs *ship*.

Synthetic training involves phrase and sentence-level material or whole passages. By providing the speech material in its linguistic context, the patient has access to semantic, contextual and topic cues. This enables the patient to use a 'top-down' language-processing approach (Lubinsky, 1986) as a compensatory strategy when receiving an incomplete message. Synthetic training is also sometimes referred to as global training (Cook, 1991). An example is the use of text following, where the patient attempts to follow and keep the place in a text read by the therapist. This is one of the first synthetic training exercises encountered by many CI recipients.

A staged competency-based auditory rehabilitation programme

Overview

The different stages of speech perception training have been described above. In Chapter 4, we emphasised the importance of beginning training at the CI recipient's current level of speech perception ability. A pre- or perilingually deafened adult with an implant is likely to have very different training needs from a postlingually deafened one. Similarly, a patient with an implant who has a long period of auditory deprivation before receiving the implant is likely to require training at a lower speech-perception level initially.

Therapists may already have access to auditory training materials published or provided by some manufacturers of cochlear implants, e.g.:

- *Nucleus 22 Channel Cochlear Implant System Rehabilitation Manual* (Mecklenberg et al., 1986)
- *Learning to Hear Again with a Cochlear Implant* (Wayner et al., 1998)
- *Auditrain* (Plant, 2001), *Hear at Home* (Plant, 2002a), *Speech Trax* (Plant, 2002c), *Syntrain* (Plant, 2002b).

In addition, a variety of training resources has been published over the years that can be adapted for auditory training for adults with cochlear implants. These include material originally written to provide training for hearing-impaired and profoundly deaf adults (Plant, 1984, 1994), exercises designed to teach speech reading (Kaplan et al., 1995) and communication strategies (Erber, 1996, 2002), exercises written to train speech perception in hearing-impaired children (Romanik, 1990), and materials written for conversation practice for teaching English as a second language (Watcyn-Jones, 2002; Watcyn-Jones and Howard-Williams, 2001, 2002). The last contain activities that are designed for interactive use.

For the clinician or therapist beginning in this field it can be a daunting and time-consuming task to source materials that provide an appropriate level of varied material for each patient. In this chapter we suggest how materials from a variety of sources can be used. In our implant programmes we have often either developed these materials further, to create additional activities, or modified them to make them more or less challenging. In some cases the original exercises have been modified to make them more relevant to CI recipients. The resources regularly used in our programme are listed below and are referred to in the training programme. They would provide a new programme with sufficient variety of task and level of difficulty to accommodate most patients. The key resource texts are:

- *Pair Work 1* (Watcyn-Jones and Howard-Williams, 2002)
- *Pair Work 2* (Watcyn-Jones, 2002)

- *Grammar Games and Activities*, Book 1 (Watcyn-Jones and Howard-Williams, 2001)
- *COMMTRAM* (Plant, 1984)
- *SYNTREX, Clinician's Handbook* and *Client's Handbook* (Plant, 1996)
- *Communication Therapy for Hearing Impaired Adults* (Erber, 1988)
- *Communication Therapy for Adults with Sensory Loss* (Erber, 1996)
- *Hearing, Vision, Communication and Older People* (Erber, 2002)
- *Nucleus 22 Channel Cochlear Implant System Rehabilitation Manual (Cochlear Manual)* (Mecklenberg et al., 1986).

To provide the therapist new to this area with a starting point, an activity is described for each stage of each level. Readers are encouraged to access the 'other suggested activities' as well as creating material of their own using local resources and materials, and using the activity as a 'design guide'. For each of the three levels of training, the therapist will find:

- overall objectives
- the rationale for, or background to, training at this level
- methods of presentation
- examples of activities.

The activities described within each level are progressively more challenging. For each exercise, a hierarchy of tasks, in increasing order of difficulty, follows a short introduction. Although the activities are provided as an example for that level of training, many of them will work at other levels, e.g. the closed-set lists for discrimination can be used as an identification task. Similarly, the material provided for identification tasks can be used for recognition practice by not allowing the patient to see the set of answers. Some exercises, e.g. text following and/or connected discourse tracking (see Exercises 2D and 3K below), can be used throughout the training programme.

The therapist should monitor the patient's progress and, if necessary, decrease the level of challenge using the suggestions provided as a guide. At the end of each exercise, sources for additional exercises, or material that can be used to generate similar activities, are listed.

In Chapter 4, the importance of addressing the CI recipient's specific hearing difficulties and goals was emphasized. Many of the exercises serve not only to improve listening and speech perception skills, but also to maximize the awareness and use of cues in conversation to enhance speech recognition. Where an auditory training exercise can be used to highlight or discuss a particular compensatory strategy, suggestions are made.

The following guidelines for presenting auditory training material may be useful:

- Sit facing the patient
- The best way to remove visual cues is to ask the patient to look down
- Use a normal voice level and natural presentation
- Initially use a slightly slower presentation rate but maintain natural rhythm
- Use very clearly articulated speech, especially at the beginning
- Pause to allow response time
- Provide positive feedback of items correctly perceived; avoid negative feedback
- Use acoustic highlighting (Estabrooks, 2001) to emphasize items missed or misperceived (i.e. emphasis, pause, stressed intonation, exaggerate feature being worked on).

Level 1: discrimination

Objective

The objective of this level of training is to teach the patient to selectively attend to different speech features or cues. The patient is required to discriminate whether two stimuli presentations are the same or different (i.e. the same stimulus presented twice or two different stimuli).

Background

Consolidating this skill is an important precursor to the next level of speech perception, i.e. identification. The ability to discriminate can be trained at a number of different levels. The patient can be trained to discriminate suprasegmental cues (such as syllable number and word stress), and segmental cues such as different vowels or consonants. Discrimination tasks can also be presented with synthetic materials, e.g. the patient can be trained to listen for the same or different sentence length or intonation. These exercises can also be used to enhance the patient's awareness of features in speech in preparation for 'text following' (see Exercise 2D, p. 119) because some patients may be able to perform 'text following' while still benefiting from training on discrimination tasks.

Method of presentation

Two stimuli are presented to the client, e.g. a monosyllabic word '*for*' and the three-syllable word '*information*'. The therapist draws the patient's attention to the feature being discriminated. In this case it is the number of syllables. The therapist identifies and reads both stimuli of the pair (auditory-alone presentation and pointing to each word as it is said) several times to allow the patient to attend to the difference(s). Finally the therapist presents two stimuli, either identical or two different ones, auditory alone with no visual indicator. The patient is required to state whether the stimuli were the same or different.

Exercise 1A: discrimination of word length

In this activity the patient is trained to listen for all components of a word. This includes detecting the difference between the word and silence, i.e. when the word finishes, listening to rhythm and paying attention to syllable number. The patient learns that, even before a word can be identified, this compensatory skill can be used to infer its identity based on the word length cues. These are important and complementary skills to speech reading.

Exercise hierarchy

Initially, the patient is presented with highly contrasting pairs such as one versus four syllables (e.g. *cat* vs *caterpillar*) and then progresses to differences of only one syllable. Asking the patient to state the number of syllables further increases task difficulty. If the patient finds the task too challenging, use stimuli with more than one contrasting feature, e.g. spectral contrast as well as syllables, or simplify the stimulus, e.g. clapping can be used – one clap versus five claps. Exercises of this type can be found in Plant (1984, Chapter 2) and Erber (2002).

Exercise 1B: discrimination of words with contrasting phonemes

This activity aims to draw the patient's attention to contrasting phonemes while the word length remains constant. As the patient is required only to discriminate whether the words are the same or different, the task is manageable by many pre- and perilingually deafened CI recipients with relatively little experience with their implant.

Exercise hierarchy

Initially, word pairs with highly contrasting phonemes are used, e.g. in the pair *'hesitate'* and *'library'*, the first word contains the unvoiced /h/, /s/ and /t/, whereas the second word contains voiced consonants, e.g. /l/, /b/ and /r/. Maximum use is made of phonetic features that CI recipients find easier to discriminate in the early post-implant period, such as voicing and manner of articulation. Initially the CI recipient may find the discrimination easier if the vowels are either highly contrasting in formant frequency or length (e.g. 'mice' vs 'load', 'bit' vs 'spice'), or occur in different positions in the word (e.g. 'cheerful' vs 'canteen'). As the exercise progresses, shorter words are used and so the patient has fewer contrasting features to assist discrimination. Pairing words with more similar features increases the task difficulty.

Suggested stimuli

- *COMMTRAM* Chapter 2 (Plant, 1984). This resource also includes exercises that isolate specifically consonant confusions in voicing, manner or place of articulation. Although the lists were created as an identification task, the material can be presented as a discrimination exercise.
- Analytika (Plant, 1994) provides a vast resource of word pairs that contrast all possible combinations of speech phonemes.

Exercise 1C: discrimination of sentence length

This activity enables discrimination to be practised with synthetic materials and can provide preparation for the 'text following' exercise below. Building on the activities in Exercises 1A and 1B, the patient will also gain experience in using word length, phonemic contrasts and temporal pattern in combination, in order to discriminate whether the two sentences are the same or different. It may also help the training of auditory memory.

Exercise hierarchy

Initially, the therapist works with one pair of sentences at a time. The first examples may contain many different features including sentence length and the number of multisyllable words and total word number in the sentence, e.g. *'cherries grow on trees'* vs *'put your empty lunchbox on the table'*. As the patient becomes more confident and experienced, sentences with more similarities can be attempted.

Suggested stimuli

- *COMMTRAM*, Chapter 2, Syllables in Sentences (Plant, 1984). This material can be presented as a discrimination or identification task.

- *Cochlear Manual* (Mecklenberg et al., 1986): analytical materials.
- *Auditory Skills Program*, Book 1 (Romanik, 1990): sentence level exercises.

Exercise 1D: discrimination of sentences with the same or different intonation

This activity gives practice at extracting this suprasegmental cue from speech by isolating it as the only distinguishing feature. In some cases the cue will be an increase in intensity created by placing emphasis on a particular word. In other cases the cue will be a change in pitch (Edgerton, 1985). The therapist can demonstrate the task by asking the patient to say each phrase, first as a statement, then as a question (e.g. 'He went to the party!' vs 'He went to the party?'). By using this progression, the patient's attention will be drawn to this feature and its role. The importance of intonation, when used to gain meaning from a partially heard message, can be explained to the patient.

Exercise hierarchy

Extremes of phrase length increase the difficulty of this task. For very short phrases the change in pitch may be contained in only the last word. Longer sentences require greater attention. The task can be made easier by exaggerating the prosodic cues.

Other suggested stimuli

- Edgerton (1985, p. 84): 'Examples of conversational phrase prosodics'. This provides examples of how intensity and pitch can be varied in four sample sentences.

Level 2: identification

Objective

This level of training aims to improve the client's ability to identify or label an auditory stimulus. This is achieved through repetitive training and the use of a set of possible alternatives. Immediate feedback is given after each response.

Rationale

The ability to identify speech at both single word and sentence level is a precursor to the ability to recognize and understand the communication intent. Where possible, stimuli should be used that are likely to have some functional value in the patient's daily life.

Method of presentation

This level of training employs closed-set tasks where the patient is provided with a target list of stimuli from which to select an answer. Training begins with familiarization, i.e. the target words or phrases are said repeatedly ('drilled'). This exposes the patient to the stimuli and allows him or her to listen for the differences. During the training, the therapist can draw the patient's attention to the distinguishing features of the stimuli or contrasts. The therapist then gives one stimulus, randomly selected from the target list, and the patient is asked to identify it. Some patients prefer to point to the matching written stimulus; others will more naturally verbalize the answer. The level of difficulty can be increased by including more items in the set and/or by selecting stimuli that have more similar phonemic properties.

The following sections provide the hierarchical steps and stimuli for identification training at word, phrase and sentence level.

Exercise 2A: identification of phonemes

Identification of consonants and vowels has been shown to be influenced by implant type, the speech processor (e.g. Dorman and Loizou, 1997) and the speech processing strategy used (Dorman, 1993; Wilson, 2000). From the consonant and vowel confusion matrices derived from single-channel CI users (Edgerton, 1985), it was clear that these patients could use voicing and manner of articulation information but could not discriminate place of articulation. This was because place information resides predominantly above 1 kHz, a frequency region not well resolved by the single-channel implant. Even with intracochlear multichannel implants, with the earlier speech-processing strategies, patients appeared to discriminate voicing and manner earlier in their implant experience and to develop skills in discriminating place of articulation later. However, since the availability of advanced combination encoder (ACE) speech-processing strategy we have noticed that CI recipients now make fewer errors and that the previous hierarchy of difficulty no longer seems to apply, i.e. some CI users are able to discriminate place of articulation relatively soon after switch-on. Postlingually deafened CI users also appear to make few vowel confusions with this strategy. For this reason, training in phoneme identification is either omitted in our programme or much reduced. For those requiring resources to consolidate these skills in pre- or perilingually deafened CI users or those with long-standing deafness, the reader is directed to the well-organized lists in *COMMTRAM* (Plant, 1984).

Exercise 2B: identification of words

Exercise 2Bi: familiar names

The aim of this exercise is to provide an achievable and highly relevant early stage task by which to introduce the skill of identification. This task employs a small set of highly familiar names of varying syllable number and word length. During this task, the greater ease of understanding of *overlearned* or highly familiar words and their usefulness in the communication situation can be discussed with the patient and family.

Exercise hierarchy

Ask the patient and family to suggest around six to eight very familiar (family) names and from these select two highly contrasting words, e.g. contrasting syllable number. Using two at a time, drill and then identify randomly selected stimuli from the pair. Add more names as the patient's skill and success level increase. However, ensure that those initially selected have highly contrasting features. Expanding the set to include the names of friends, pets, relatives or work associates can increase task difficulty.

Exercise 2Bii: months of the year

The aim of this activity is to extend identification skills. The speech stimuli are the months of the year and the set size increases the potential for confusion. The patient learns to attend to and use both syllable and spectral information.

Exercise hierarchy

Begin by drilling and random identification from highly contrasting pairs, e.g. March and September. Use combinations of these pairs to form sets of four then six, adding progressively more pairs until the patient can work with all twelve.

Exercise 2Biii: weekdays

Although the target set is smaller than that in Exercise 2Bii, the difficulty is increased because all but one of the stimuli have two syllables and all contain the same final syllable 'day'.

Exercise hierarchy

Begin with the sets of three words with highly contrasting phonemes. Point out the contrasts (syllables, vowel length) to the patient, e.g. the set contains one three-syllable word 'Saturday', 'Monday' begins with a short vowel in contrast to the long vowel in 'Tuesday'. Once the patient can discriminate from sets of three, use the set of all the days of the week.

Exercise 2Biv: numbers up to twenty-one

This task presents greater difficulty because many of the words are single syllable and some share the same vowel and/or consonant (e.g. five/nine, two/ten, fifteen/sixteen). The stimuli have high incidence in daily life increasing their functional relevance.

Steps

- Begin with sets of four numbers with highly contrasting features. Including numbers with more than one syllable will reduce the difficulty initially. Next provide larger set sizes but retain contrasting phonemes and stimuli of different syllable length.
- Provide stimuli of the same syllable length to increase the difficulty further. Potential confusions (e.g. two/ten and fifteen/sixteen) may need to be introduced last.
- Increase the task difficulty by using ordinal numbers. i.e. first, sixteenth, as the addition of the relatively short high-frequency 'th' can make this particularly challenging. Alternatively, increase the set size.

Suggested stimuli

Other highly familiar closed sets, which may be used in this way, include fruits and colours.

Exercise 2C: identification of phrases and sentences

Exercise 2Ci: identification of responses to common questions

This task uses everyday questions that increase the task relevance (e.g. 'Do you have children?', 'Are you spending Christmas at home?').

Exercise hierarchy

The *patient* asks the therapist a question that has a 'yes' or 'no' answer, i.e. a closed set of two. The patient must ascertain whether the therapist replied 'yes' or 'no'. Next, a set of possible replies, each with a qualifier, is provided (e.g. Q: 'Can you drive a car?' A: 'Yes, I enjoy driving.' 'No, I'd rather take public transport.'). The patient must identify which of the replies was used. Increasing the length and complexity of the reply can be used to vary the degree of difficulty. The patient can use the initial (yes/no) response together with the sentence length to assist identification.

Suggested stimuli

- *Pair Work 1* (Watcyn-Jones and Howard-Williams, 2002), Exercise 21, 'Daily Life', p. 71. This is a list of questions beginning 'Do you . . . ?' with a set of four possible replies ('Yes, I always', 'I often', 'I sometimes', 'No, I never'). The exercise can be used as described above.
- *Grammar Games and Activities*, Book 1 (Watcyn-Jones and Howard-Williams, 2001), Exercise 24 'Life style surveys' (p. 76). This exercise provides several sets of questions beginning 'Do you?' (e.g. 'Do you enjoy shopping?'). There are six possible answers, e.g. 'No, hardly ever', 'Yes, always'. This exercise can be used as described above, or the therapist and patient can reverse roles.

Exercise 2Cii: identification of missing words

The patient is presented with a list of incomplete sentences and, for each, a set of words or phrases that would complete them. All of the items in the set would be semantically appropriate. The patient is required to listen to a sentence spoken by the therapist and, using segmental or suprasegmental features of speech, identify which word or phrase, from the set of possibilities, was used to complete the sentence.

Exercise hierarchy

The task difficulty is increased by varying the availability of contrasting features, set size, position of missing word in the sentence, length of sentence, familiarity of words and number of missing words. The task can be extended by either adding words or including items with less contrast. The material in this exercise can be used at the recognition level by not providing the set of possibilities. In this case it can be used to discuss the value of semantics (e.g. word relations and word order) and the underlying *linguistic framework* as well as *context* as compensatory strategies.

Suggested stimuli

- *SYNTREX*, Clinician's Handbook (Plant, 1996), Chapter 8 'Fill in the gap sentences', pp. 113–121. Twenty sentences are listed with two to four alternative words. Alternative words with differing levels of predictability are provided. Selection of a less predictable word to fill the gap will make this task more challenging for the listener.

Exercise 2Ciii: identification of word combinations

The requirement to identify two or three components, spoken by the therapist, each selected from a *different* closed set, e.g. date and month, increases the challenge. The use of previously rehearsed items in Exercises 2Bii and 2Biv means that the material is familiar and the patient has a sense of building on previous skills. The high occurrence of the stimuli (dates) in everyday conversation increases the task relevance. This material can be used to discuss value of 'limited set questions' as a compensatory strategy. The therapist may insert the word 'of' between the stimuli if desired.

Exercise hierarchy

* Two-word combinations are selected from each of two closed sets, e.g. 4th June, 17th of March. Alternatively, a two-word combination can be constructed using the standard card set, e.g. six (of) hearts, or numbers and shapes, e.g. four circles
* Three-word combinations are selected from the following three closed sets, i.e. day, date, month
* The task difficulty can be increased by varying the order of presentation, e.g. Wednesday, January (the) 9th.

Other suggested stimuli

* In an alternative task, the therapist presents items from a closed set of everyday items (a litre of milk, loaf of bread, local stamp) and their cost. The patient repeats back and uses knowledge of the cost of items to give an appropriate reply.
* The therapist describes a person in terms of height, hair and eye colour, e.g. tall (with) brown hair and blue eyes. The target sets should be defined beforehand.
* *Auditory Skills Program*, Book 1 (Romanik, 1990) contains examples at a lower language level if required.

Exercise 2Civ: identification of sentences

In this task the patient must listen to whole sentences. The patient is presented with a set of sentences, and then the therapist presents one sentence and the patient must identify it from the set. During this activity, the therapist may discuss how listening for *key words* can be used as a compensatory strategy.

Exercise hierarchy

The task begins with just two sentences, which is then extended by two as the patient gains skill and confidence. Using sentences of a similar length and word number will extend the difficulty of the task. Sentences with words of different syllable number or frequency content will make the task easier. The use of topics of high relevance or interest such as work-related phrases, common questions or 'things people say about wearing their cochlear implant' may make the task more interesting/relevant for the patient.

   Other suggested stimuli

- *COMMTRAM* (Plant, 1984), 'Topic centred sentences' pp. 190–4, Training lists 1–10
- *Cochlear Manual* (Mecklenberg et al., 1986): over-learned related sentences
- Composed set of sentences relevant to the patient's situation.

Exercise 2D: paragraph or text following

In this identification task, the whole paragraph is used. The client employs skills acquired in identifying words or groups of words. The exercise reinforces the use of suprasegmental (rhythm, word length) and prosodic cues in speech (intonation). It encourages the patient to consider whether the speech perceived makes sense (semantics) as well as whether it matches the words to which he or she is pointing. The task encourages the patient to pay attention to the whole phrase. This is a good exercise to use for a 'warm-up' at the start of an auditory training session. It enables the patient to tune into the speaker's voice rather than attending to visual cues.

Exercise hierarchy

The therapist or support person reads the paragraph, stopping at times. The patient must follow the text and is required to identify or repeat the last word spoken. The following methods for increasing difficulty can be employed:

- Choose a text with a simple everyday language style. Use a slow presentation rate with stops at predictable boundaries.
- Increase the speed of presentation, and use random stopping points such as the middle of a sentence.
- Increase the task difficulty by employing a faster presentation rate or a signal degraded in some way, such as the therapist moving while speaking or use of low-level background noise such as a radio.

* Use more complex texts with unfamiliar vocabulary.

Suggested stimuli

* Text from magazines of high interest to the patient
* Newspaper editorials
* Extracts from testimonials or books written by other CI recipients
* Recipe books
* *SYNTREX*, Clinician's Handbook (Plant, 1996), 'Questions and answers', pp. 13–30. Although this passage was designed to be used as a comprehension task, the short passages can be used for following text.

Level 3: recognition and comprehension

Objective

This is to improve the patient's ability to recognize and comprehend auditory information, both with and without contextual clues.

Rationale

The patient uses the auditory signal to recognize the verbal stimulus in the open-set condition (i.e. without having any familiar or rehearsed set to choose from). In most of the following tasks, as the words are not nonsense words and are generally vocabulary that the patient will already know, the task involves some degree of comprehension because memory, vocabulary, knowledge about sentence structure and experience may be employed by the patient to help 'fill in' the missing information.

Method of presentation

In earlier stages of this level, topic-limiting clues are provided or the therapist may give feedback about correct words, making this a 'semi-open-set' task. In some tasks the therapist reads the stimulus and the patient is simply asked to repeat it verbatim. Some tasks are interactive, requiring the patient both to listen to a sentence or utterance and to provide information or carry out an instruction. As the client becomes more skilled and confident, the emphasis moves away from listening to and repetition of every word towards responses that demonstrate that the patient is listening for the message or meaning. In all tasks at this level, there is scope for the client to use strategies to clarify the stimulus, and this aspect is clearly built in to some of the exercises. As the patient's speech recognition skills improve, there is less emphasis on purely information transfer and more on the social interaction aspects of speech perception.

Exercise 3A: missing information – high familiarity

Method 1

This exercise is an extension of Exercise 2Cii. The main difference is that the patient is not provided a set of possible answers from which to complete the sentence and must rely on context to do so. The patient is presented with a set of everyday sentences from which key words are missing (e.g. The young ___ helped the ___ lady to cross the ___). The therapist presents the complete sentence. The patient attempts to repeat it. The use of common everyday phrases or overlearned phrases such as proverbs (Plant, 1984) can be used to discuss the value of 'linguistic structure', 'word order', 'prediction' and 'word association' as compensatory strategies during this exercise.

Exercise hierarchy

Initially, the missing words should be highly predictable. Increasing the number of missing words and using less predictable words or phrases to complete the sentence increases the difficulty. If the task is too difficult, additional key words can be presented.

Suggested stimuli

- In the activity SENT IDENT (Erber, 1996, 2002) the patient is presented (auditory alone) with a sentence, which he or she attempts to repeat verbatim. If the patient does not correctly repeat the sentence, the therapist repeats it up to four times using commonly used repair strategies until it is repeated with 100% accuracy. Each repetition uses a different form of repair in a hierarchical fashion, i.e. repetition, repetition with emphasis/elongation, key word given with visual cue, whole phrase repeated with visual cues. By providing only a segment of each sentence this can be adapted into a 'missing information' task.

Method 2

This adaptive assessment method provides the patient with the opportunity to be, alternately, the listener and the speaker. It provides the therapist with the opportunity to assess the client's comprehension from both their understanding of the stimulus and their responses to the therapist's questions.

Exercise hierarchy

The therapist and client begin with sets of incomplete information in which the missing information is different and complementary. The therapist and patient attempt to complete the missing information by alternately asking each other a question, e.g. the information could be a person's personal details. An example of such an exercise can be found in Exercise 7 'Four people' of Grammar Games and Activities, Book 1 (Watcyn-Jones and Howard-Williams, 2001).

When the missing information belongs to a specific set, such as numbers, colours, animals, dates, cities or countries, girls names, vehicles, etc. the topic cue makes the task easier, providing a link between the easier closed-set exercises and the more challenging open-set tasks that follow. The set of target answers can be expanded to include less common alternatives to increase difficulty.

Other suggested stimuli

- *Grammar Games and Activities*, Book 1 (Watcyn-Jones and Howard-Williams, 2001). In the activity 'What are the missing numbers?' on page 45 the information is arranged into a numbered matrix. The participants ask for the content of specific squares in the grid, e.g. what number is in square 4B? This exercise provides an opportunity to discuss the use of *limited choice questions* to assist speech recognition.
- *Grammar Games and Activities*, Book 1 (Watcyn-Jones and Howard-Williams, 2001): 'Fill in the missing dates', p. 46.

Exercise 3B: phrases with highly predictive and familiar answer format

The patient uses both the context and prior knowledge about how this information is usually phrased to assist with comprehension. This increases the likelihood of success at recognition level, providing an ideal early stage exercise. The task builds on the number identification skills of Exercise 2Biv. It provides further opportunity to practise clarification strategies, and to discuss *word relations* and *frequent pairing*, e.g. 'quarter past', as compensatory strategies to aid speech recognition.

Exercise 3Bi: what time?

Method

The therapist presents, one by one, a list of specific times of day which the CI user attempts to repeat. Alternately, the patient asks the therapist at what time he or she usually performs various everyday activities using a list of prepared prompts. The therapist creates a suitable answer. The therapist can indicate either by repetition or using various clarification strategies, whether the time was correct, e.g. 'yes, that's correct', 'not quarter *past* 7 (quarter *to* seven)' or ' listen again to the number'.

Try to avoid giving the client negative feedback, because this may be perceived as criticism, when the individual is trying hard to work on a speech perception task. An alternative would be to respond, 'You thought I said, "quarter *past* seven", I actually said, "quarter *to* seven"; this gives the client the chance to hear the small contrast for him- or herself.

Exercise hierarchy

Initially a standard format is used such as ten minutes to/past seven. Using alternative formats (such as '7:10', or '5 to 6', or 'at 10 past 7 in the evening' or '12 o'clock', 'midday' and 'noon', or 'fourteen hundred hours') can increase or decrease the degree of redundancy/difficulty.

Exercise 3B ii: dates

Exercise hierarchy

As above, the therapist gives specific dates and the client attempts to repeat them. The patient either repeats or records the date. Initially, a standard date format is used '14th April 1950'. Later, the format can be varied to encourage the person to listen to *all* of the information, e.g. 'In 1923 on the 23rd day of July'. This builds on the discrimination skills learned in Exercises 2Bii and 2Biv.

Other suggested stimuli

- Family birthdays or anniversaries
- Dates of birth of famous people
- *Grammar Games and Activities*, Book 1 (Watcyn-Jones and Howard-Williams, 2001), 'A day in the life of . . .', p. 51, could provide a template for your patient to perform an activity with a family member or support person in which the patient asks the communication partner the time of day when various everyday activities were performed

Exercise 3C: extracting relevant information

The patient may have reached the stage of attending to longer utterances and be able to *extract the relevant information* from a sentence. In this exercise, the questions asked by the patient will limit the answer provided by the communication partner in both content and structure. The patient asks the therapist questions about his or her ideal home. The therapist creates suitable answers. The patient asks a variety of questions to build up a complete picture, e.g. how many rooms does it have? Does it have a garden? Is it one storey or two? Is it inland or by the sea? The task difficulty is related to the size of the set to which the answers are limited and the extent to which the question allows the patient to anticipate the vocabulary in the answer. The patient attempts to recognize and record the information. The patient is encouraged to use a variety of clarification strategies to check that the information has been correctly perceived. This activity provides the patient with an introduction to the use of context, predictability, limited-choice questions and requests for specific information as compensatory strategies. The patient can also be encouraged to use clarification strategies.

Exercise hierarchy

The therapist manipulates the complexity of the information supplied, from concise and predictable to an answer embedded in a sentence. Altering the length and difficulty of the vocabulary in the sentence and the position of the information within it can increase the level of difficulty.

This activity can also be an interactive exercise. The therapist and CI patient each have a description of a different house for sale (sources include local newspapers and real estate brochures). The therapist and patient alternately ask each other questions about the features of the house and record the information. The level of difficulty for the patient would then be dictated by elements of unpredictability in the question format, e.g. 'How many bathrooms does the house have?', 'Does it have space for one or two cars?' and 'Is it close to the city centre?'.

Other suggested stimuli

- *Grammar Games and Activities*, Book 1 (Watcyn-Jones and Howard-Williams, 2001), Exercise 7, pp. 47–8, 'Four people'.
- *Pair Work 1* (Watcyn-Jones and Howard-Williams, 2002), Exercise 17, p. 64 'For Sale'. This exercise invites the client to ask questions to fill in the gaps of a newspaper advertisement.
- *Pair Work 1* (Watcyn-Jones, 2002), Exercise 10, p. 55, 'Renting a Holiday Home'. The client is required to prepare questions to find out more about a newspaper advertisement. The therapist then answers the questions in a role-play scenario.
- *Grammar Games and Activities*, Book 1 (Watcyn-Jones and Howard-Williams, 2001), Exercise 23, pp. 74–5 'Biographies'. This exercise contains two biographies with different and complementary missing information.

- Descriptions of cars for sale in a local newspaper.
- The ASQUE procedure (Erber, 1988) demonstrates to the patient how the received response can be made more or less predictable by the way that the preceding turn is phrased. Questions and statements are grouped according to the type of response that would be elicited (e.g. yes/no, fixed choice, limited set, general). These can be used to generate discussion between the patient and therapist about how different types of question can affect the intelligibility of the answer.

Exercise 3D: sentence recognition

Exercise 3Di: topic-related sentence recognition

Method 1

In this activity the patient is informed of the topic of the material (e.g. sports, children) and is asked to listen to and repeat the related sentences that follow. The patient is encouraged to use semantic context, topic clues and associated words to guess any part of the sentence that was missed or only partially heard. It can be helpful to provide the patient with a list of potential clarification strategies to refer to during this exercise.

Exercise hierarchy

When this exercise is first introduced, the therapist may stay well within the topic boundaries and use highly contextual sentences, i.e. many of the words in the sentence are related to the topic. As the patient's level of skill and confidence increases, less familiar vocabulary, less related material, use of common nouns and longer utterances can be used. The last will also extend the patient's auditory memory.

A staged approach can be used to encourage the patient to use repair strategies. Initially the therapist can assist by repeating and rephrasing together with positively reinforcing all attempts by the patient to initiate repairs. Gradually the therapist encourages the patient to initiate repairs by not always providing feedback when misunderstanding occurs. With the confident patient, the therapist may occasionally use an unrelated sentence to provide an opportunity for the patient to detect an irrelevant utterance or change of topic.

Other suggested stimuli

- *COMMTRAM* (Plant, 1984), 'Topic centred sentences' (e.g. 'Things people say about meals and food') can be a useful resource or starting point to which the therapist may create additional sentences with more local content.

Other suggested topics

Pets
Health
At work
Telephone banking
Local sights
Sentences related to the patient's workplace or hobby.

Method 2

The patient is provided with a picture or drawing of a scene which provides
the topic context and vocabulary. The therapist and the patient may discuss
the picture first to prime the patient with the relevant vocabulary. The
therapist can use the picture in a number of ways

• Make statements about the picture, which the patient then repeats, e.g.
  'The dentist is wearing glasses', 'The boy is opening his mouth'.
• Ask the patient questions about the picture, e.g. 'How many bottles of
  wine are on the picnic rug?', 'How many people are having a picnic?'.

In a more challenging version, the patient is asked to memorize as much
detail as possible before either repeating statements or asking questions
about the picture without having it in front of him or her.

Other suggested stimuli

• Pictures from magazines, newspapers and client-relevant publications
• Diagrams from the patient speech processor handbook.

Exercise 3Dii: context-related sentence recognition

This activity is similar to the one above but the patient is provided with a
situation clue. In this activity the patient is informed of the situation context
(e.g. phrases you might hear in hospital) and is asked to listen to and repeat
the sentences that follow. This task may present more challenge, because the
vocabulary may be more wide ranging.

Other suggested stimuli

• *Cochlear Manual* (Mecklenberg et al., 1986): Context-related sentences
• *Pair Work 1* (Watcyn-Jones and Howard-Williams, 2002), Exercise 15, p. 62
  'The kitchen cupboard' and Exercise 18, p. 66 'Richard's student room'.

Exercise 3E: topic-related interactive exercises

Working within the boundaries of a topic, the patient's recognition/ comprehension skills can be extended by engaging the patient in topic-related dialogue with the therapist. The interactive nature of this exercise also provides the opportunity for the patient to practise communication strategies (see Chapters 6 and 7). The patient can use context and prediction to anticipate the vocabulary in the answer and is encouraged to listen for key words or those that convey the most meaning. The application of this skill to daily life can be discussed.

Exercise 3Ei: newspaper advertisements

The following is a role-playing exercise. The patient is supplied with an advertisement from a newspaper (suggestions: pets for sale, cars, furniture). The therapist plays the role of the person selling. The patient responds to the advertisement by asking the therapist for more information and then negotiating a price. The patient can be supplied with the prompts and/or make up questions of his or her own.

Exercise hierarchy

The difficulty of the answers generated by the therapist can be adjusted to meet the skills of the patient. The therapist may try short answers to reduce redundancy, introduce new vocabulary and reply to a question with another question.

Exercise 3Eii: booking an apartment for a weekend

Exercise hierarchy

The patient is given a brief brochure description of a holiday apartment. The patient's task is to ask the therapist questions about the apartment and make a booking. The therapist generates appropriate answers that the patient may repeat or write down. The therapist can increase the difficulty by replying with questions, e.g. 'How many people will be coming?', or by embedding the answers within sentences of increasing length. This encourages the patient to listen to *all* of the information.

Other suggested stimuli

- Local newspaper 'for sale' or 'shared accommodation' section.
- Holiday brochures.

- Newspaper travel and accommodation section.
- *Grammar Games and Activities*, Book 1 (Watcyn-Jones and Howard-Williams, 2001), Activity 49, 'House share', p. 120.
- The therapist and patient may ask one another questions about the town or city where they were born/grew up.
- TOPICON (Erber, 1996, 2002) is a conversation practice procedure in which the CI recipient or therapist may select a topic from a given list (e.g. saving money, dogs, today's news) and then conduct a brief conversation on the topic for around 5 minutes. After the conversation participants may discuss the fluency of conversation, the number of breakdowns, the ability to anticipate vocabulary and the CI recipient's confidence to participate, for example. A guide and form for assessing the fluency of the conversation are provided.

Exercise 3F: overlearned phrases – no topic clue

When the patient is able to work within a topic with confidence, overlearned sentences or sentences that follow a predictable, highly familiar pattern can be employed gently to move the patient away from reliance on topic and/or situation clues. The therapist may confirm any words correctly repeated. The patient is encouraged to use correctly repeated words to guess what the phrase might be.

Exercise hierarchy

The therapist reads highly familiar phrases to the patient who then repeats the phrase. In the second stage a question and answer format is used with very familiar questions. Initially the therapist asks the questions. As the patient's skill and confidence increase, the patient may ask the questions. The therapist can make the task easier initially by giving short and highly predictable answers.

Suggested stimuli

- *COMMTRAM* (Plant, 1984), p. 170, questions about things that you like and pp. 171-4 'The Helen Test' which contains questions such as 'what is the opposite of hot?'

Exercise 3G: sentences on different topics with clue words

Using unfamiliar topics and vocabulary increases the difficulty in this activity. This task will usually engage the patient in clarification strategies. During this exercise, compensatory strategies such listening for key words, listening for meaning rather than exact recall and word association can be discussed.

Exercise hierarchy

Before each stimulus the patient is given a single clue word. Depending on the patient's ability the key word may be with or without lip-reading. The therapist says the related sentence. The patient is asked to repeat it. Depending on the patient's skill level, the therapist may acknowledge those words that are correct. The patient is encouraged to make use of clarification strategies such as 'please speak more slowly', 'please say that another way', 'what was the word after . . .' and 'please spell that word'.

Other suggested stimuli

- *Cochlear Manual* (Mecklenberg et al., 1986): unrelated sentences with clue words.
- Contingent stimulus response pairs (Erber, 1996, 2002) provide a list of topic clue and sentence pairs (e.g. topic: 'Illnesses'; stimulus: 'Everyone in our family has a bad cold'). The therapist may use this material as a speech recognition task initially. The therapist may then go on to use the material for communication therapy as intended by the author, i.e. to encourage the patient to predict what a frequent communication partner is likely to say in response (in the example above 'I hope you will all feel better soon'). This exercise demonstrates the compensatory strategy of how one person's utterance affects what the other person is likely to say.

Exercise 3H: following instructions

This activity provides the patient with practice at comprehension for meaning rather than exact recall, listening to and remembering instructions, and coping with multiple instructions. The degree of challenge can be manipulated by increasing the length and/or the number of instructions. The patient is encouraged to use clarification strategies, e.g. 'Did you say X or Y?'

Examples of following instruction include instructions to perform common tasks such as following directions from one place to another on a local map, following a recipe, drawing objects in a predetermined pattern or sequence, completing a form or performing a simple relaxation exercise, for example.

Other suggested stimuli

- The therapist may instruct the patient on how to do or make something, e.g. make a pancake or pot of tea, decorate a Christmas tree or walk to the clinic from the centre of the city. The number of instructions given in each utterance varies the difficulty. The patient repeats back the instructions. The predictive value of successive sentences as a compensatory strategy can be discussed.

- *Pair Work 2* (Watcyn-Jones, 2002) 'Complete the drawing', Exercises 10 and 13, pp. 58 and 64
- *Grammar Games and Activities*, Book 1 (Watcyn-Jones and Howard-Williams, 2001), Activity 29, 'Trace the route', pp. 84–5
- *Grammar Games and Activities*, Book 1 (Watcyn-Jones and Howard-Williams, 2001), Activity 11, 'Up, down, left, right'
- *Pair Work 1* (Watcyn-Jones and Howard-Williams, 2002), 'Where's the tourist information office?' Exercise 20, p. 69
- *Pair Work 1* (Watcyn-Jones and Howard-Williams, 2002), 'Following instructions', Exercises 13 and 19, pp. 59 and 67
- *Pair Work 2* (Watcyn-Jones, 2002), 'Read and remember: Four families', Exercise 28, p. 94
- *SYNTREX*, Clinician's Handbook (Plant 1996), pp. 76–83, 'Map reading provides both maps and questions about directions'
- *SYNTREX* Clinician's Handbook (Plant, 1996) 'Questions and instructions: List 7' p. 65, provides the client with context for the listening task; however, the speech discrimination task requires a high degree of fine phonemic discrimination, e.g. the therapist instructs the client to 'Draw a line under the 3' and the client has a choice of '3, bee, etc.'.

Exercise 3J: simulated conversation practice

Rationale

In this activity the patient and conversation partner are engaged in a simulated conversation using a half-script. A most effective tool of this kind is QUEST?AR (Erber, 1988). The conversation revolves around a place that the clinician has been to, either of the clinician's own choosing or using a suggestion from the list supplied. The *patient* is provided with a half-script – a prepared series of inter-related 'Wh' questions to find out about the visit. The therapist or support person supplies an answer. The patient may be asked to repeat the answer to ensure that it has been understood. Initially the therapist generates answers that are highly predictable and short. As the patient gains competence, the task difficulty is increased by the use of less familiar vocabulary, longer utterances and less predictable answers.

This activity can be used to draw the patient's attention to a number of compensatory strategies, including informed guessing, topic, conversational intent and prediction. It provides the patient with the opportunity to direct the conversation, which appears to build confidence in many of our CI recipients. One of QUEST?AR's most valuable aspects is that it provides many natural opportunities for the patient to use clarification strategies. A similar exercise can be performed using a half-script to arrange to go to a movie/

picnic/sporting activity (example questions might be: 'When shall we go?', 'What sort of movie shall we see?', 'Would you like an old movie or a new release?', 'Should we invite any friends along?').

Other suggested stimuli

- *Pair Work 2* (Watcyn-Jones, 2002), 'Complete the dialogues', Exercise 39, p. 108.

Exercise 3K: connected speech or connected discourse tracking

Rationale

This task, described as 'tracking' by DeFilippo and Scott (1978), can be used to document an individual's progress in recognizing and comprehending connected speech. The therapist reads a text, segment by segment, and the patient is required to repeat it verbatim. It allows the patient to take advantage of rhythm, stress and syntax cues. More recently it has been developed as a tool to train patients in coping strategies for daily conversational management (Owens and Raggio, 1987). Indirectly, this exercise provides a 'safe' environment in which to practise assertive and problem-solving behaviours and to learn the value of providing feedback to the speaker. It encourages the patient to attend to auditory stimuli and to take an active part in managing conversation breakdown.

It can be used at any time in the patient's rehabilitation once the patient is successful at the recognition level. The patient's performance can be recorded and compared across sessions. If the reader wishes to use this procedure primarily as a measurement tool, the original published (shorter) directives may be more appropriate.

Background

One of the greatest values in this exercise is the problem-solving approach applied when the patient does not understand all or part of the segment. In the original method, the therapist or trainer assumed responsibility for communication breakdown, in both initiating when to offer direction and choosing which particular strategy, or clarification method, to apply, e.g. repeating a word or reading more slowly. Owens and Telleen (1981) developed this tool further so that it could also be used to teach coping skills for conversation breakdown in the real world. In their approach, it was the listener's responsibility to decide when and how to solve the breakdown. If the listener could not repeat the segment, the reader waited for directives as to which strategy to apply.

Method

The exercise may be used to offer variety in recognition tasks and to train CI patients in resolving communication difficulties, rather than as a means of quantifying progress. The strategies shown in Table 5.1 reflect wording that may be acceptable in daily life. The requests incorporate strategies that elderly CI recipients and those with English as a second language, who may demonstrate slower speed of processing, have found beneficial in this task. Similar strategies are discussed in Owens and Raggio (1987), Kaplan, Bally and Garretson (1985) and Erber (1988). As suggested by Owens and Telleen (1981), the role of talker and listener can be reversed.

Information for the patient

The patient is provided with the topic and, if desired, a list of the proper nouns in a story or text. A list of clarification strategies is placed in front of the patient.

Familiarization

In the practice session both auditory and visual (speech reading) cues may be used to train the patient in the task. If the patient finds this very difficult, allowing him or her to read through the text in the first one or two sessions can allow him or her to complete the training. A slower speed of delivery may be used initially. At first the therapist may present short three- to five-word chunks in a meaningful segment, whenever possible. Therefore, some texts may require editing before presentation in order for longer sentences to be broken down into meaningful segments. These are increased as the patient demonstrates increased skill and confidence levels. The patient is encouraged to repeat back all words heard, even if it is only part of the segment and to guess as much as possible. This is crucial to the aspect of learning the value of feedback. In this practice session the therapist can demonstrate each of the strategies as the opportunity arises. The patient can then be encouraged to try each of the strategies themselves.

Table 5.2 contains a summary of therapist responses, based on those of Owens and Raggio (1987).

The advantages and disadvantages of some strategies can provide a useful discussion with the patient. Spelling may be the only way a patient may understand an unfamiliar word or proper noun. This is time-consuming and the patient may forget the first few letters with words over five letters long. Patients should be encouraged to write down the spelling as they resolve the word so that they are not trying to juggle too many cognitive tasks at the same time. Repetition of the whole segment provides the context but it is time-consuming

Table 5.1 Strategies

Please say that again
Please repeat the (first/last) word
Please repeat the first/last part
Could you say that another way?
Could you use a different word?
Please use a louder voice
Please use a shorter phrase
Please speak more slowly
Please spell that word

Table 5.2 Therapist responses

Patient response	Therapist action
Segment repeated correctly	Nod, and go on to next segment
Segment repeated partially but correct	Fill in the rest of the segment
Segment only partially correct	Repeat entire segment, perhaps stress the incorrect words
None of segment correct	Shake head, wait for directive
Patient does not respond	Wait for directive

and generally less acceptable to the general public. Therefore, we generally steer patients away from using this option too frequently. The task can be used to demonstrate that use of an alternative word, instead of several repetitions, can sometimes repair the breakdown faster.

If the text has been modified (e.g. following a request to rephrase), this becomes the target text as long as the meaning is the same. After the familiarization period, the task is performed for around three consecutive minutes on average. If a quantitative measure is required, the patient's score is the number of words repeated per minute (total number of words divided by total number of minutes). If the clock is stopped while the communication breakdown is resolved, the number of times the clock is stopped could also be noted.

Suggested stimuli

Texts that are of general interest, simple in vocabulary, culturally sensitive and written in everyday language appear to work best. Owens and Raggio (1987) report that descriptive paragraphs were found to be more difficult than narrative ones. Graded readers and text written to teach English as a second language can provide appropriate level text because the language complexity is not too great and there is sufficient text for several sessions. It should also ideally be interesting to the patient and cater to the patient's language proficiency.

Exercise 3L: passage comprehension

Rationale

The main value of this exercise is that it encourages listening for meaning and encourages the patient to concentrate on key words rather than listening to every word.

Method

The therapist reads a short passage out loud to the patient (auditory alone). The therapist checks the patient's comprehension of the passage by asking questions about it. Initially the passage should contain everyday vocabulary, be short and contain simple sentence structures. As the patient's skill increases, the task can be made more challenging using longer passages, less common vocabulary and unfamiliar material.

Other suggested stimuli

Newspaper editorials
Excepts from magazines
Movie reviews
Sections from the CI recipient's own speech processor handbook.

References

Cook BO (1991) Testing and rehabilitation of cochlear implant patients at the department of Audiology, Ssonderjukhuset, Stockholm. In: Cooper H (ed) Cochlear Implants: A Practical Guide. London: Whurr Publishers, 240–50.

Cooper H (1991) Training and rehabilitation for cochlear implant users. In: Cooper H (ed.), Cochlear Implants: A practical guide. London: Whurr Publishers, 219–39

DeFilippo CL, Scott, BL (1978) A method for training and evaluating the reception of ongoing speech. Journal of the Acoustical Society of America 63: 1186–92

Dorman MF (1993) Speech perception by adults. In: Tyler RS (ed.), Cochlear Implants: Audiological foundations. San Diego, CA: Singular Publishing Group, 1993: 145–90

Dorman MF, Loizou PC (1997) Changes in speech intelligibility as a function of time and signal processing strategy for an Ineraid patient fitted with continuous interleaved sampling (CIS) processors. Ear and Hearing 18: 147–55

Edgerton B (1985) Rehabilitation and training of postlingually deaf adult cochlear implant patients. Seminars in Hearing 6: 65–88

Erber NP (1982) Auditory Training. Washington DC: A.G. Bell Association for the Deaf.

Erber NP (1988) Communication Therapy for Hearing Impaired Adults. Abbotsford: Clavis.

Erber NP (1996) Communication Therapy for Adults with Sensory Loss, 2nd edn. Melbourne: Clavis

Erber NP (2002) Hearing, Vision, Communication, and Older People. Melbourne: Clavis

Estabrooks W (2001) What is Auditory-Verbal Therapy (AVT)? In: Estabrooks W (ed), 50 FAQs about AVT: 50 Frequently asked Questions about Auditory-Verbal Therapy. Toronto: Learning to Listen Foundation, 2–8.

Kaplan G, Bally S J, Garretson C (1995) Speechreading – a way to improve understanding. Washington DC: Clerc Books

Lubinsky J (1986) Choosing aural rehabilitation directions: suggestions from a model of information processing. Journal of the Academy of Rehabilitative Audiology 19: 27–41

Mecklenberg DJ, Dowell RC, Jenison VW (1986) Nucleus 22 Channel Cochlear Implant System Rehabilitation Manual. Cochlear Ltd

Owens E, Raggio M (1987) The UCSF tracking procedure for evaluation and training of speech perception by hearing-impaired adults. Journal of Speech and Hearing Disorders 52: 120–8

Owens E, Telleen CC (1981) Tracking as an aural rehabilitation process. Journal of the Academy of Rehabilitative Audiology 14: 259–73

Parkinson AJ, Arcaroli J, Staller SJ, Arndt PL, Cosgriff MD, Ebinger K (2001) The Nucleus 24 Contour cochlear implant system: adult clinical trial results. Poster presented at The American Academy of Audiology, San Diego, CA, 2001

Plant G (1984) COMMTRAM. A Communication Training Program for Profoundly Deaf Adults. Sydney: National Acoustics Laboratories

Plant G (1996) SYNTREX : Clinician's Handbook and Client's Handbook. Somerville, MA: The Hearing Rehabilitation Foundation

Plant G (1994) Analytika. Analytic testing and training lists. Somerville, MA: The Hearing Rehabilitation Foundation

Plant G (2001) Auditrain. Innsbruck, Austria: MED-EL

Plant G (2002a) Hear at Home: A home training programme. Innsbruck, Austria: MED-EL

Plant G (2002b) Syntrain. Innsbruck, Austria: MED-EL

Plant G (2002c) Speech Trax. Innsbruck, Austria: MED-EL

Romanik S (1990) Auditory Skills Program, Book 1. NSW: Department of School Education

Tye-Murray N (1993) Aural rehabilitation and patient management. In: Tyler RS (ed.), Cochlear Implants: Audiological foundations. San Diego, CA: Singular Publishing Group, 87–145

Watcyn-Jones P (2002) Pair Work 2. Harlow: Penguin English Photocopiables, Pearson Education Ltd

Watcyn-Jones P, Howard-Williams D (2001) Grammar Games and Activities Book 1. Harlow: Penguin English Photocopiables, Pearson Education Ltd

Watcyn-Jones P, Howard-Williams D (2002) Pair Work 1. Harlow: Penguin English Photocopiables, Pearson Education Ltd

Wayner DS, Abrahamson JE, Casterton J (1998) Learning to Hear Again with a Cochlear Implant. Hear Again, Inc., 1200 Madison Ave, Austin, TX: Advanced Bionics

Wilson B (2000) Strategies for representing speech information with cochlear implants. In: Niparko JK (ed.), Cochlear Implants: Principles and practices. Philadelphia, PA: Lippincott Williams & Wilkins, 129–69

Chapter 6
Aural rehabilitation following cochlear implantation: forming an intervention plan

KAREN PEDLEY AND ELLEN GILES

In Chapter 4 the advantages of a holistic, client-focused, goal-based rehabilitation programme were described. The intervention plan is a summary of the client's goals, the skills required to meet those goals and the areas of training that may help the cochlear implant (CI) recipient to develop those skills that are not present or are inadequate. The therapist may draw on all areas of therapy – auditory training, conversation and communication therapy – to assist the CI recipient to achieve his or her goals. A tool such as COSI in Appendix 13 (Dillon et al., 1997) is recommended. Specialist areas such as telephone training and training in the optimum use of assistive listening devices are covered in Chapters 10 and 11 of this book. The therapist may consider the following areas and questions when identifying the training needs:

What level of speech perception does the CI recipient demonstrate and does the CI recipient pay attention to all of the available cues in conversation?

When the client is encouraged to guess during speech perception training, which of the following cues does the patient use:

- Topic cues
- Situational cues, e.g. where the conversation takes place, a person's job
- Knowledge of the preceding conversation
- Linguistic cues, e.g. frequent pairing, word order, grammar rules, relations between words, contingent pairs (i.e. how a response is related to what was previously said)
- Speaker cues (local colloquialisms, shared experiences).

Erber (1988) suggests that a hearing-impaired person who uses all contextual cues achieves greater conversational fluency and provides a detailed discussion of this area for the interested reader.

Which communication situations does the CI recipient find difficult?

Which communication strategies does the CI recipient demonstrate in these difficult listening environments and what areas would benefit from communication therapy? Communication therapy develops the patient's awareness of, and practical experience with, one or more of the following skill areas:

- Conversation tactics including turn-taking, eye contact, being an 'active listener' and use of non-verbal cues (Brooks and Cleaver, 1989).
- Environmental management strategies or 'constructive strategies' (Tye-Murray et al., 1993) such as reducing background noise or avoiding shadows on the speaker's face.
- Conversational partner management skills, e.g. requesting the speaker to speak more slowly or keep the head still while speaking.
- Anticipatory strategies, or strategies for *preventing* communication breakdown, e.g. anticipating the possible content of the interaction (Tye-Murray, 1992) or anticipating the typical sequence of a conversation (Erber, 1988, 1996, 2002).
- Metacommunication skills, i.e. 'the ability to think about communication and talk about it' (Erber, 1988).
- Assertive responses.
- Conversational repair strategies (see below).
- Lip-reading skills.

The social–interactional elements of communication therapy and suggested exercises/activities for building skills in this domain are described in detail in Chapter 7. The proportion of time spent on each will be determined by the individual needs of each patient. Tye-Murray et al. (1993) advocate the use of self-assessment methods to establish the extent of the functional use of communication strategies by the patient and/or the frequent communication partner (FCP). In the daily diary method described, the FCP is asked 'What did you do when your relative did not understand your message?' and is presented with a checklist of possible strategies.

How frequently does conversation breakdown occur, i.e. mishearing, misunderstanding, corrections, rephrasing for example? Does the CI recipient and/or the FCP demonstrate a range of repair strategies?

Repair strategies aim to increase the likelihood that the communication and/or reply will be understood. Increasing the CI recipient's and the FCP's awareness and use of conversational repair strategies can improve conversational flow and, hence, the perception of both the CI recipient and

FCP that the conversation was successful. Conversational repair strategies have been described in detail by several authors (e.g. Erber, 1988, 1996, 2002). In Tye-Murray et al. (1993) useful summaries of strategies and examples of their use are listed.

Repair strategies include attempts by the FCP to manipulate the choice of language to improve intelligibility of his or her utterance. Examples are:

- elaborating the message to provide redundancy
- repeating a segment
- indicating the topic
- simplifying the message to draw attention to key words or reduce the need for auditory memory
- message organization to avoid verbosity, generality, irrelevancies (for examples, see Tye-Murray and Witt, 1997)
- using more common words.

The therapist can consider whether a limited or wide range of strategies is evident and if the FCP uses strategies spontaneously or only in response to requests by the CI patient.

Some CI patients will demonstrate the need for significant work in this area such as those frequently feigning understanding or not responding at all when the conversation breaks down. Where the hearing loss was sudden, the CI patient (and FCP) may have had less time to develop repair strategies. The therapist should determine the CI patient's awareness of available strategies. Does the CI patient make general (e.g. 'Sorry, what was that?') or specific requests to clarify information missed or partially heard? Does he or she use clarification strategies such as requests for repetition of all or part of the message (e.g. 'What was the last word, again?', 'Did you say . . .?'), and requests for alternative words or phrases (e.g. 'Could you please say that a different way' or 'Please use shorter sentences')?

Does the CI patient tend to use open-ended questions or attempt to phrase the question to make the reply easier to understand/more predictable? Examples of question styles that may improve intelligibility include 'limited choice questions', i.e. questions that limit the response set to a few possible alternatives (e.g. 'what colour is his new car?'), forced choice questions (e.g. 'would you prefer tea or coffee?') or requests for specific information (e.g. 'what suburb do you live in?'). For further discussion of conversation therapy strategies that can shape the conversation turn, the reader is referred to Erber (1988, 1996, 2002) and Lind (2004).

There are a number of methods to establish whether both the CI recipient and the significant other/FCP are using a variety of repair strategies. This may be achieved informally through participation in conversation, by observing the CI patient and FCP in conversation or during interactive activities such as connected discourse tracking (CDT) and QUEST?AR as described in Chapter 7. Alternatively, a more structured assessment could be used such as a self-assessment questionnaire for the FCP (Tye-Murray et al., 1993) or a proforma for recording repair types and turns taken in repair (Lind, 2004). To enable the therapist to pay attention to this aspect, it can be helpful to video the session, and observe the client working with the FCP or another therapist. For the therapist wishing to focus on this aspect of communication training, a three-stage model of formal instruction, guided learning and real-world practice is described in Tye-Murray and Witt (1997).

Do the desired goals/training areas indicate the need for intervention by other professionals?

When working through the intervention plan, consider whether other support or therapy could contribute towards the CI recipient's goals. These could include, for example, a speech and language therapist (see Chapter 8), the CI team psychologist, a specialist in vocational training (see Chapter 9) or a lifestyle counsellor (relaxation or stress management). The timing and availability of supporting intervention will be important considerations.

Example intervention plans

Case 1: Mr S

Background

Mr S has a progressive postlingual hearing loss. Retaining his work position is a high priority. Before implantation, his position was in jeopardy as a result of severe hearing difficulties. Mr S finds some work colleagues, especially those with accents, and soft female voices difficult to follow. He feels comfortable making requests of his work colleagues to change the way that they speak but admits that this frequently does not improve the communication. Mr S finds some sounds in the work area very distracting since obtaining a CI. Mr S has increasingly avoided telephone use, finding it very stressful. He prefers other methods of communication within the work place, which is not always appreciated by work colleagues.

Broad goal

Improve communication with work colleagues.

Specific goals

- Understand speech better in daily meetings in open plan office
- Improve acoustics of his immediate work area
- Increase understanding of the implant limitations among his work colleagues
- Improve accuracy of understanding internal phone messages.

Skills areas	Speech perception	Use of cues	Communication strategies	Equipment	Other
Areas of competence	Good open-set speech recognition in quiet with own family	Uses linguistic cues well	Uses assertive requests of speaker well, but does not always identify what the problem is	Use of alternative methods such as fax, email	
		Recognizes phone tones			
Areas for training	Perception of soft/female voices	Use of key words	Anticipatory strategies	Use of processor settings to enhance soft speech	Increase understanding of CI within the workplace
	Perception of degraded speech in quiet	Use of speaker and situation cues	Environment management strategies addressing speaker characteristics	Use of direct input device for phone and inbuilt telecoil	
	Perception of speech in competing speech situations		Telephone tactics	Use of FM system for meetings	
	Perception of speech over the phone				

Therapy plan

- Practice with CDT, with clear, conversational, accented and soft speech, and speech in multi-talker babble (MTB)
- Auditory training with sentences relevant to situation and speaker
- Auditory training with patients own work-related sentences in quiet, then in MTB

- Perception of sentences with progressively softer speech using speech processor setting to enhance, e.g. sensitivity, 'whisper', customized gain settings
- Practise extracting key information using exercises involving 'exchange of information' and instruction following tasks in quiet and in MTB
- Anticipatory strategies such as obtaining agenda, minute of meetings
- Compensatory strategies: sitting beside minute taker, setting up room for meeting
- Exploration of patient's work environment and ways to improve it
- Increase awareness of speaker characteristics and applying existing assertive skills to this area
- Closed-set discrimination of work-related vocabulary by phone
- Role-play of frequently occurring work situations in quiet, in MTB, by phone
- Provide information session to work colleagues (see below)
- Exploring ways to use FM system with conference microphone transmitter in group meetings

Case 2: Miss P

Background

Miss P is a congenitally deaf young adult working in a retail environment. She has been moderate-to-severely hearing impaired all her life with very little hearing above 2 kHz. Post-implant, Miss P has some closed-set speech perception abilities but no open-set speech recognition. Miss P has always found communication at work stressful, but is very aware of how environmental aspects affect comprehension and makes appropriate assertive requests in this regard. She is aware that she does not always respond to her name or various auditory signals at work, and sometimes does not respond appropriately to her colleague's feelings in communications, who subsequently become embarrassed. Her work colleagues become impatient because they are often asked to repeat the whole utterance several times.

Broad goal

To enhance communication with her work colleagues.

Specific goals

- To enhance the perception of speech with lip-reading
- To be more responsive to feelings of work colleagues
- To improve the clarity of her own speech, if possible

- To enhance understanding of the implant capabilities/limitations among her work colleagues
- To reduce danger from inability to recognize alarms
- To be more involved in break-time conversation at work.

Skills areas	Speech perception	Use of cues	Communication strategies	Equipment	Other
Areas of competence	Good discrimination		Environmental strategies	Optimizing use of sensitivity and volume	
	Some identification of closed-set speech		Assertive requests	Use of telecoil	
Areas for training	Improve perception of high frequency speech cues	Use of all cues to enhance closed-set recognition	Repair strategies	Use of lapel microphone	Work place demonstration of the CI device and its limitations
	Enhance closed-set recognition		Conversational partner management		Speech clarity
	Enhance use of auditory cues as an aid to speech reading				Recognition of alarms at work
	Practice in recognizing emotional cues in speech				

Therapy plan

- Analytical training with high-frequency speech sounds
- Closed-set identification with stimuli selected for presence of low- and high-frequency cues
- Text following to enhance recognition of high frequencies in speech
- Closed-set auditory training with work-related vocabulary
- Closed-set sentence recognition with topic-related and context-related sentences
- Sentence training with visual cues to enhance use of topic and all context cues

- Listening practice with passages or sentences using different emotional cues
- QUEST?AR to enhance repair strategies
- Conversation partner management exercises
- Interactive exercises/role-playing with visual cues and lapel microphone
- Workplace information session
- Auditory training (with workplace personnel if possible) to enhance recognition of fire and other workplace alarms and auditory signals
- Referral to speech and language therapist for assessment re potential for improvement in speech clarity.

Case 3: Mrs B

Background

Mrs B is a 78-year-old CI recipient with a postlingual progressive hearing loss who received the implant in her seventh decade after a very long period of profound loss, during which many environmental cues were inaudible. Mrs B demonstrates good understanding of common sentences without lip-reading but accuracy deteriorates significantly when the speed of presentation is increased even marginally. She resides independently but in a complex with support from specialized staff. The complex is beside a busy road. Family members visit frequently. All those caring for Mrs B report that Mrs B often feigns understanding and that they are often unsure how much has been understood. Mrs B tends to avoid communication with the support staff, especially medical and paramedical staff, because she reports that they tend to shout or over-exaggerate facial movements when talking with her. Mrs B finds that the road noise reduces speech understanding but does not understand how to use the speech processor features to improve this aspect.

Broad goal

Improve communication with all those who visit regularly.

Specific goals

- Increase Mrs B's confidence in, and control of, conversation
- Reduce communication breakdown
- Develop more appropriate communication tactics in the support staff.

Skills areas	Speech perception	Use of cues	Communi-cation strategies	Equipment	Other
Areas of competence	Speech perception for normal conversational speech	Uses situational and topic context well	Good use of conversation strategies and visual cues	Maintenance and battery management	
		Listens for key words			
Areas for training	Speech perception for fast speech	Use of speaker cues	Awareness and use of repair strategies by both family, patient and support staff	Improve independence with speech processor controls	Increase understanding about the CI with residential support staff
			Environmental issues	Use of lapel microphone	

Therapy plan

- In-service training session for support staff, especially use of clear speech and repair strategies
- Targeted training of environmental cues especially alarms
- CDT for progressively faster speech – listening for meaning
- CDT for encouraging use of repair strategies by both patient and FCPs
- Trial of speech processor settings and ALDs to reduce road noise
- QUEST?AR with family (and support staff, if willing) for clarification strategy training
- ASQUE-type exercises with patient to encourage use of more specific questions with paramedics
- Recognition of sentences related to specific speaker types (GP, podiatrist, etc.)
- Anticipatory strategy training
- Training in assertive requests for improving the speaker characteristics of FCPs
- Assessment and management of Mrs B's communication environment
- Instruction in use of and trial of lapel microphone for some visitors that are hard to follow

Case 4: Mr G

Background

Mr G is a postlingually deafened CI patient. Mr G demonstrates a very high level of open-set speech perception but the score is significantly reduced by the addition of competing noise. He had been unable to use the phone for 4 years before implantation. When he used the telephone with the hearing aid, his family frequently became impatient, particularly if he was unable to hear a phrase after many repetitions. Mr G developed the habit of writing notes before he made a call. Some family members were much easier to understand than others but Mr G is not sure why. Mr G reported most success when he knew the topic of conversation. In face-to-face communication Mr G gets frustrated when a communication breakdown occurs. He knows a range of communication strategies, but does not feel comfortable about applying them in daily situations.

Broad goal

To be able to use repair strategies in a range of situations: on the telephone, at home and work.

Specific goals

- To be able to telephone his family who live interstate.
- To feel comfortable about asking for help when he gets into communi-cation difficulties with his family, friends and colleagues.

Skills areas	Speech perception	Use of cues	Communi-cation strategies	Equipment	Other
Areas of competence	Good open-set speech recognition in quiet	Uses prediction and semantic cues Recognizes phone tones	Anticipatory strategies	Use of telecoil	
Areas for training	Identifying the caller	Following changes of topic	Clarification strategies	Obtain and learn to use adapter for direct input	

(continued)

Skills areas	Speech perception	Use of cues	Communication strategies	Equipment	Other
Areas for training	Perception of degraded speech and speech in noise		Conversational partner management	Mobile phones	
	Perception of speech by telephone		Making assertive requests		

Therapy plan

- Practise with CDT, with degraded speech (soft speech, speech in noise)
- Obtain telephone adapter; practise answering phone/connection routine
- Text following over the telephone using moderate and faster rates of speech and speakers with different accents
- Recognition of unrelated sentences with word topic cue face-to-face and by phone
- Identifying names by phone – closed set, open set
- Awareness of clarification strategies and practice in their use with single scripted conversation, and role-play obtaining information, face-to-face, then by phone
- Awareness of speaker characteristics and their effects, practice in assertive requests of the speaker
- Invite to a psychosocial workshop to explore use of communication strategies and assertive techniques
- Training in making assertive requests of therapist, phone buddy, family members, work colleagues
- Instruction in use of direct input phone device
- CI patient to arrange trial of different models of mobile phones

Workplace/residential care information sessions

With the trend to offer implantation to patients with more residual hearing, therapists may encounter CI recipients in the workplace with increasing frequency, i.e. patients have not reached the point where they have needed to give up work. A holistic approach may include providing an in-service training/information session in the patient's workplace to inform, help dispel misconceptions and encourage appropriate communication behaviour. The opportunity could also be used for further exploration of ways to improve the environment where applicable.

Such a session was provided to the employees of a supermarket where a prelingually hard-of-hearing CI recipient worked. It soon became apparent that the co-workers expected her to return to work with normal hearing and speech! The session focused on the benefits and limitations of the implant. It was emphasized that the implant would not 'cure' the person's hearing or speech problems. Appropriate communication strategies were demonstrated, the need for lip-reading emphasized and allowances for the CI recipient tiring quickly were discussed. The co-workers were encouraged to help in identifying and localizing environmental sounds. A demonstration 'head' showing visually how the implanted electrode array responds to sound is always well received at such demonstrations. The CI recipient reported numerous positive outcomes of the presentation. These included a reduction in her anxiety about returning to work, facilitation of communication with her colleagues and acceleration in her awareness of environmental cues at her work place. When a similar session is offered at a residential care environment, issues concerning care and maintenance of the device can also be covered.

Conclusion

A range of therapies is required to offer individuals the best support with their cochlear implant. These include auditory training, conversation and communication therapy, use of assistive devices and use of psychosocial workshops to address the needs of the client and to enable skills to be transferred from the clinic into everyday situations.

References

Brooks DN, Cleaver V (1989) Communication training. In: Brooks DN (ed.), Adult Aural Rehabilitation. London: Chapman & Hall, 170–86

Dillon H, James A, Ginis J (1997) Client Orientated Scale of Improvement (COSI) and its relationship to several other measures of benifit and satisfaction provided by hearing aids. Journal of American Academy of Audiology 8: 27–43

Erber NP (1988) Communication Therapy for Hearing Impaired Adults. Abbotsford: Clavis.

Erber NP (1996) Communication Therapy for Adults with Sensory Loss, 2nd edn. Melbourne: Clavis

Erber NP (2002) Hearing, Vision, Communication, and Older People. Melbourne: Clavis

Lind C (2004) Conversation therapy following cochlear implantation. In: Pedley K, Lind C, Hunt P (eds), Adult Aural Rehabilitation – A guide for CI professionals. Sydney: Cochlear Ltd, in press

Tye-Murray N (1992) Preparing for communication interactions: the value of anticipatory strategies for adults with hearing impairment. Journal of Speech and Hearing Research 35: 430–35.

Tye-Murray N, Witt S (1997) Communication strategies training. Seminars in Hearing 18: 153–65

Tye-Murray N, Knutson JF, Lemke JH (1993) Assessment of communication strategies use: questionnaires and daily diaries. Seminars in Hearing 14: 388–51

Chapter 7
Social–interactional elements of communication therapy for adult cochlear implant recipients

CHRISTOPHER LIND AND LISA DYER

> Hearing impairment has been extensively studied from a pathophysiological and psychoacoustic standpoint. Procedures have been designed to cure or compensate this sensory limitation. However, relatively little attention has been given until now to the key factor of rehabilitation outcome, that is, the meaning people ascribe to hearing impairment. Being human involves trying to make sense of events. Having a hearing loss is a major life event for most people . . . people devote much more effort to try to adjust to the problem of a spoiled social identity and social exclusion than to try to restore their hearing and communication abilities.
>
> Hetú (1996, p. 22)

This chapter is aimed at health professionals: audiologists, speech pathologists, teachers and others who work with individuals who have hearing impairments. It concentrates on aural rehabilitation techniques because they may provide assistance to adults in individual therapy sessions. With few changes these exercises may also be adapted to suit younger cochlear implant (CI) recipients and group rehabilitation programmes. The material in this chapter has been influenced primarily by the work of Erber (1996, 2002), Kaplan et al. (1995) and Trychin (Trychin and Boone, 1987; Trychin, 1988), whose models of intervention have provided an emphasis on the interactional aspects of conversation, assertiveness and the role of the conversation partner. Texts by Gagné and Tye-Murray (1994), Kricos and Lesner (1995) and Tye-Murray (1998) have also informed the rehabilitation model presented, and interested readers are guided to their works. Those who are familiar with these authors will note their influence throughout this chapter in the design and content of the work presented here. Those who are not familiar with these texts are urged to refer to them for their important theoretical discussions and useful practical exercises.

Everyday conversation is a socially motivated event. Conversation is used to organize and inform, to interact and relate. It is a complex activity, demanding of participants' attention and often requiring exquisite planning and timing skills, yet adults indulge in it successfully and seemingly without effort many times a day. People converse for all manner of reasons, and in each and every conversation the way in which they talk to each other is influenced by the purpose of the interaction, and the shared knowledge among participants as well as the physical setting in which it takes place. Successful conversation requires adults to address these issues in each and every setting.

Adults who have acquired hearing losses (and who subsequently may have received a cochlear implant or hearing aid) may find that conversational difficulties arise as a result of the impact of the hearing impairment on the particular interaction. Further, these may have adverse social consequences both for them and for the people to whom they are talking. Intervention aims to minimize the effects of the hearing impairment on the conduct of everyday conversation by bringing elements of conversational behaviour under the conscious control of the CI recipient with the acquired hearing impairment and his or her daily conversation partner(s). This programme is based on the development of a hierarchy of abilities by which adults with acquired hearing impairment may (re-)establish successful or fluent daily conversation. The hierarchy involves:

- bringing under the CI recipient's awareness the factors within everyday conversation that may adversely influence the success of a conversation
- increasing the CI recipient's awareness of the aspects of the environment that might be changed to improve the success of a conversation and the strategies by which they may be changed
- developing the CI recipient's ability to gain the communication partner's understanding and assistance in undertaking these changes.

In this social–interactional approach, *activity limitation* or *disability* is seen as the consequence of the interaction between the individual and his or her communication partner, the content and process of the conversation and the (physical and social) environment. This approach incorporates methods that are designed to acknowledge the complexity and variability of everyday spoken communication. The following are the guiding principles:

- Therapy is client centred and situation specific: CI recipients are seen within the context of their daily lives and the nature of each conversation in which they are involved will define the needs of the individual in that communication. In the first instance therapy is designed to address the predictable elements of each of these situations, and then to apply them as potential solutions to a wide range of instances of everyday conversation.

- Therapy is flexible enough to meet the expressed everyday communication needs of the CI recipient. Intervention programmes are designed to address the issues raised by the patient, clinical exercises are fine-tuned to those needs, and the outcome of intervention is measured by reference to these stated needs of the CI recipient.

- The goals of therapy are mutually negotiated between CI recipient and clinician, and regularly reviewed in consultation with the patient. The relationship between therapy goals and the CI recipient's desired outcomes is made overt. CI recipients are encouraged to take part in the planning of the therapy process and to take responsibility for the structure and outcome of the therapy, the sequence of therapy events, and the onset and cessation of therapy.

- Therapy brings aspects of everyday conversational behaviour under the conscious control of the CI recipient. The clinical task is to create informed and well-equipped CI recipients who can consciously assess and address previously difficult situations successfully. Therapy should take into account the CI recipient's beliefs, and knowledge about and attitudes towards both the hearing impairment and his or her involvement in everyday conversation.

- Therapy is based on strategy rather than massed practice alone. Therapy is designed to address the CI patient's attitudes, beliefs and knowledge about his or her communication skills, and to allow him or her to assist in the practice of conversation behaviours.

- Therapy incorporates the communication partners that the CI recipient wishes to involve in the therapy. We encourage the attendance of the CI recipient's *significant other* (SO) or *frequent communication partner* (FCP) to either individual or group programmes to facilitate this process further. All conversation requires substantial cooperation between participants (this is particularly pertinent to those who are in frequent communication with the hearing-impaired CI recipient). Involving frequent (or indeed infrequent) conversation partners in the therapy process highlights the need for understanding and cooperation in order to minimize the difficulties that arise in conversation from the hearing impairment.

- Therapy may be conducted as individual and group programmes. This rehabilitation model is amenable to both individual and group instruction. Although this model highlights the very individual nature of interaction and the need to address issues within the context of each CI recipient's daily life, there is a deal of face validity in group programmes.

Aspects of everyday conversation

People converse in order to be understood by others. Participants in conversation respond to both the content and the intent of others' turns, often referred to as the *transactional* and *interactional* elements of a speaker's turn (Pichora-Fuller et al., 1998). Different instances of conversation give different weight and form to these transactional and interactional elements. Contrast the purpose(s) of a chat 'over the back fence' with a neighbour with the talk that may occur at a job interview. A CI recipient's concerns about conversations occurring at a social gathering are likely to be different from the concerns arising from a business meeting, a medical appointment or an interaction with a shop assistant in a busy shopping centre.

Successful conversation is based on the establishment and maintenance of shared understanding between participants in each conversation. Participants develop a mutual understanding with respect to a particular topic during a conversation. Each turn is interpreted within context of talk that that has led up to it, and simultaneously shapes the subsequent context. For conversations to work, participants need not only to interpret each turn in relation to the prior context, but also to make their understanding clear and overt, i.e. they need to acknowledge their understanding of the prior turn for the purposes of the current conversation. This acknowledgment occurs with each participant taking the next turn (Clark and Wilkes-Gibbs, 1986; Clark and Schaefer, 1987). However, there are instances in almost every conversation when one or other participant may find that he or she has not understood some or all of the content in one of the previous turns. It is the responsibility of that participant to identify that he or she is unclear about something that has been said, caused, possibly, by a mishearing, misunderstanding or misinterpretation of something that has been said. This is a normal and 'unremarkable' part of conversation. To do it successfully participants must monitor their own and others' speaking turns very closely and identify (relatively immediately) when these mishaps occur.

Everyday conversation includes many instances of these mishaps, and they tend to be resolved easily and without disruption to the flow of the conversation. These mishaps tend to give rise to a commonly occurring sequence of turns aimed at resolving or repairing the breakdown. The repair sequences after a mishap or breakdown may be initiated by either participant and subsequently (re-)solved by either participant. However, if for any reason the occurrence of these sequences dominates the conversation, it is possible that one or more of the people involved in the conversation may view it as sufficiently unsuccessful to lose interest and even terminate it. The quick and efficient management and resolution of these breakdown-and-repair sequences is critical to the perception of conversational success. The social–interactional consequences of their occurrence and the manner in which they may be best dealt with in a particular conversation are the major foci of this therapy approach.

Metacommunication

The aim of this intervention is to bring aspects of conversation behaviour under the individual's conscious awareness and control; however, most people are, to a greater or lesser extent, naïve communicators. For effective discussion of conversational behaviour, it is important both for the clinician to have a grasp of the elements of conversation that may most readily influence CI recipients' conversational success, and for the CI recipient to be able to discuss these matters. Within the context of this intervention model, 'metacommunication' describes people's ability to talk about talking. The person with good metacommunication skills is able to discuss conversation and has the ability to identify and comment on characteristics of his or her own communication needs as well as the conversational characteristics of the communication partner, the environment and/or the message. This CI recipient can identify the daily life situations in which conversation is successful, and alternatively can also identify sources of conversational failure and its underlying causes. By contrast, the CI recipient with poorer metacommunication skills is often aware of the situations in which trouble arises, but is unable to analyse much of the detail of those situations. CI recipients with good metacommunication skills tend to move more easily through the social–interactive rehabilitation process. The clinician who is aware of the CI patient's metacommunication abilities may more efficiently programme rehabilitation activities to meet the individual's conversation needs.

Conversation is a cooperative enterprise, and everybody has the right to enjoy the conversations in which they participate. This involves establishing and maintaining one's own rights to achieve one's own conversational goals while maintaining other people's rights to achieve their desired goals in the conversation. It is important that each participant feel comfortable with acting assertively to establish these communication goals; however, many people misperceive assertiveness as aggression. The idea of taking steps overtly to manage the conversation is foreign to them, although it is part of almost every daily spoken interaction. It is a part of an assertiveness or *effective communication* therapy approach to let people know one's needs. It remains a problem that people with the best intentions but poor metacommunication skills may not be able to change their speech and their language characteristics to meet another's needs. By contrast, there are communication partners who are cooperative and capable of changing their communication behaviour, but who need to be directed towards the strategies that will assist the CI recipient best. These people are the focus of this chapter.

Managing the physical environment

Many rehabilitation programmes have addressed the management of the physical environment in which conversations take place by reference to hearing tactics or environmental tactics and readers are encouraged to consult work in these areas for some excellent therapy approaches. Very often the aim of environmental tactics work is to raise CI recipients' awareness of the potentially adverse effects of the three common issues: lighting, noise and distance. Useful work on environmental tactics can be found in Exercises 8, 9 and 10 in Kaplan et al. (1995, pp. 66-9). These exercises, addressing the environmental conditions in several different settings, provide excellent structured attention to the various influences of the environment on access to conversation. They allow the clinician and CI recipient to address issues about how a space might be arranged to suit oneself, and the important factors in choosing the best or most strategic set-up for communication in each particular setting. Following up the Kaplan et al. (1995) exercises it is useful to have people address their own home, work or other environment along these same lines. They may draw a floor plan of a particular room or space in which they converse regularly and apply the principles from previous exercises to this environment. Once CI recipients have tackled a number of specific environments (including their own) it is useful to have them create a list of problems. At this point, CI recipients can develop and discuss a set of strategies that they might use based on the commonalities among the situations with which they have been presented. At the end of this the aim is for CI recipients to end up with a small number of pertinent tactics that work for them over a time and across an array of circumstances.

The exercises that appear in this chapter addressing the physical environment aim to complement the work of these authors by considering the actions that CI recipients may need to take in a social context. They address the manner by which CI recipients may ask for, prompt or otherwise initiate these changes. Although many of the straight environmental issues are easily and readily dealt with, CI recipients will need to consider how best to communicate these conversational and environmental needs to others and how comfortable they feel in doing so. Many will say that they do not feel comfortable asking others to meet their (quite genuine) needs. This matter of assertiveness warrants substantial attention and will be dealt with more directly in a later section of this chapter. However, it is insufficient to have the CI recipient understand how environmental tactics may be best managed while not equipping them with the confidence to address the issues in daily life. The complexity of these situations needs to be addressed with respect to the interpersonal issues as well as a myriad of social and cultural issues. With guidance, CI recipients can identify the salient issues with respect to their interactions with others that form the basis for discussing aspects of assertiveness. This provides an opportunity to discuss with CI recipients which style feels most comfortable and to have the strategies well rehearsed.

Working with the communication partner

The perception of success (or otherwise) in a conversation influences all participants, and communication disruption or breakdown may bring into question the social communicative competence of one or all of them. Conversational success is seen here ultimately as an outcome of mutually shared responsibility, and in order for this shared responsibility to occur the communication partner may need to be guided to the situation-specific actions that may make conversation successful. As such, the inclusion of the communication partner as an active and equal partner in the therapy can be critical to the success of the process. This changes the emphasis in rehabilitation from the processing of language as information flow to the conducting of conversation as interaction. Although the communication partner may be able to assist in establishing successful communication patterns, they may not, without guidance, always know when assistance is needed or how to go about this. As well as bringing various conversational behaviours under the CI recipient's conscious control it is useful for the CI recipient to be able to enlist the cooperation of the communication partner.

The aim of an effective communication approach is to develop the CI recipient's ability to enlist the understanding and cooperation of the conversation partner and to explore with them the most efficient way of getting one's message across. Conversation success is a mutually addressed and negotiated outcome. It requires all participants to work towards it.

Although successful conversation is negotiated among participants in ALL conversations, the change to everyday conversation behaviours required to meet the needs of the patient with an acquired hearing loss will be based in part on informing the conversation partner(s) of the manner in which they need to communicate. To achieve this goal the CI recipient needs to be aware of the elements of the conversation that may be addressed and the manner in which they can be altered with a request for assistance. The focus on the role of the communication partner in this approach to rehabilitation is based on three points:

1. If the communication partner is aware of the CI recipient's communication needs he or she are more likely to respond.
2. Being aware of the nature of the problem does not assume that the person will know how to respond to it.
3. All communication about the hearing loss, however brief, must be couched in assertive language (i.e. without apportioning blame or expressing guilt for communicative breakdown).

These tactics are designed to inform the communication partner of the way(s) that they may take their portion of the responsibility to overcome the current communication difficulty. This is achieved by (1) incorporating into their speech/language behaviour the tactics that the CI recipient indicates will be most likely to be successful and (2) sharing the responsibility not to let breakdowns go unattended. These ideals reflect the individual as a reasonable adult, and that the conversation is being conducted on an equal footing. The clinician may discuss with the CI recipient how to put across to the 'reasonable' communication partner in order to optimize the likelihood of cooperation.

Clinical exercises in social–interactional aspects of communication therapy

Set out in the remainder of this chapter and in Appendix 5 are activities that have been used by the authors to address the social–interactional aspects of acquired hearing impairment and the communication difficulties that arise from them. These exercises are designed to include:

- a brief general written introduction
- a verbal introduction by the clinician concerning the way in which a particular exercise might address the CI recipient's needs
- the body of the exercise

- a discussion of the purposes and the outcomes of the exercise for the CI recipient.

These exercises are designed to increase awareness of the issues that underpin successful interaction. The manner in which the clinician uses each exercise will depend on the CI recipient's stated needs and understanding of conversation that he or she brings to therapy. These exercises allow CI recipients to address their concerns in the light of everyday contexts. The exercises follow a sequence that underpins the idea of bringing social interactional aspects of daily conversation under the conscious control of the CI recipient and their important/frequent conversation partners. This simple sequence:

- identifies the issues of the conversation that contribute to communication breakdown, and which may be manipulated
- addresses the tactics by which these might be overcome
- addresses the manner in which the tactics may be used and frames the interactional aspects of the request
- evaluates the outcome of the interactional aspects of the strategy.

Environmental tactics

Exercise 1: 'Tactics for the eye and ear'

In this exercise 10 common communication difficulties are presented and the CI recipient is asked to identify a range of possible solutions for each problem that will allow the communication goal to be achieved (or at least approximated). Emphasis in this exercise is placed primarily on finding various solutions to environmental matters (e.g. lighting, distance and noise). Although the CI recipient may offer a practical and appropriate solution to some or all of these potential problems, discussion is aimed at developing an understanding of a range of possible responses that may be suited to different situations. To apply these requires lateral thinking and once practised will enable the CI recipient to act quickly to implement the strategies. During this exercise it has been useful to incorporate discussion about how each of the strategies to overcome these problems may be/has been addressed in a particular setting or with particular people. This allows the introduction of the social–interactional elements of these tactics that are required to implement them successfully.

It is important to note that often people will be concerned that they have achieved the 'correct answer' in response to issues such as those raised in this exercise. In this (and indeed in all of the exercises in this chapter), it is necessary to dissuade CI recipients of the notion that there is a right or correct answer. The range of influences on a particular conversation may require a range of potential responses. No one response will always apply, and the decisions that underpin each response are useful points of discussion also.

Speaker and message characteristics

Exercise 2: 'Identifying characteristics of the speaker and the message'

This exercise follows the general design of the previous exercise. It provides a list of conversation behaviours that may be problematic for the CI recipient, and asks him or her to identify whether each may be a *helpful* or *unhelpful* speaker characteristic. Those listed as unhelpful characteristics may then be categorized by whether or not they are amenable to change, and thus whether they may be reasonably attempted by the CI recipient. To bring conversational behaviours under the CI recipient's conscious control, a CI recipient needs to be overtly aware of the speaker characteristics that best suit him or her in each/any situation. Although it is impractical to discuss EVERY communication setting or conversation partner, it is reasonable to approach this topic with a few clear exemplars. The strategies that most readily apply to a particular communication partner or situation divide into two groups: (1) those that manipulate the linguistic structure of one's own turn in order to influence the structure and/or content of the response, and (2) those that make overt the request for a change in the message. These strategies have been discussed elsewhere (see Erber, 1996, 2002; Erber and Lind, 1994; Tye-Murray, 1994, 1998; Tye-Murray and Schum, 1994; Lind, 2004).

It is essential to the shared responsibility of communication that the CI recipient accurately identifies the elements of the speaker and message impacting successful communication. This activity assists the CI recipient to understand and develop the analytical skills required to assess the conversation partner's interaction (e.g. rate of speech, the use of jargon, accent or reduced visual cues) into its component parts and clearly identify the positive and negative influences of each. This exercise provides an opportunity to discuss the factors that they may be able to manipulate and those that they must accept (and thus rely on other strategies to accommodate the communication impairment). As the activity requires CI recipients to reflect on their own recent communication partners, it provides authentic and valuable outcomes pertinent to their own experiences. The identification of unhelpful characteristics and the challenge to consider possible changes and how these may be implemented provides the CI recipient with tools to take to future interactions with the speaker/situation identified and to generalize to other communication situations.

Communication as a two-way process

Exercise 3: 'Elements of a conversation'

In this exercise CI recipients have an opportunity to apply their knowledge of everyday conversation, to identify the elements that may influence interaction in a range of everyday settings, and then to discuss the success or otherwise of these conversations given the range of positive or negative influences that they have identified. The CI recipient is encouraged not only to identify the positive and negative factors but also to consider achievable solutions, to trial these solutions, and to reflect and evaluate their effectiveness. The anticipatory nature of this exercise has benefit in reducing the potential anxiety associated with certain communications, which in turn increases the chance of more successful interactions. Interested readers are directed to Kaplan et al. (1995) and Tye-Murray (1992) for more detail on the importance of anticipatory tactics.

Assertiveness in communication

Exercise 4: 'Reactions to communication breakdown'

Often it is apparent in clinic that, although CI recipients are very conscious of the effects on them of conversation difficulties, they pay less attention to how this affects others. Participants share equal responsibility for conversational success. If a conversational breakdown occurs, both people will have a reaction to it. The clinician needs to discuss with the CI recipient a broader perspective, which brings the communication partner into consideration in every conversation. This activity extends the previous exercise by drawing the focus away from the sources of conversational difficulty and towards participants' responses to them. In this activity the CI recipient is asked to address the manner in which participants' reactions to conversation breakdown or difficulty may arise. The CI recipient is asked to analyse these responses with respect to the setting, and the purpose of communication, as well as participants' reactions to the problem. Finally they are asked to provide a possible solution to the difficulty. The CI recipient is asked to undertake this analysis with respect to one, two or three specific situations.

This offers an opportunity to relate conversation difficulty to its emotional and interpersonal consequences and particularly to emphasize the emotional response of the communication partner. It is the authors' experience that CI recipients often become so anxious about their own performance that they lose sight of the impact of conversation problems on the people with whom they are speaking. From this the CI recipient may assess the degree of acceptance of hearing loss achieved and the impact of this on assertive use of repairs and environmental manipulation.

Exercise 5: 'Getting what you want from a conversation'

Assertiveness is encapsulated in the maintenance of one's rights and interests while respecting the rights and interests of others. It is built on people treating their communication partners as equals, and the absence of apportioning blame or guilt (e.g. for conversation failure) that are not or cannot be reasonably identified as one individual's responsibility. Assertiveness may clearly be distinguished from passive and aggressive behaviours, the former arising when one subjugates one's own rights for another's and the latter when one ignores or lessens the importance of others' rights by comparison with their own. A passive attitude often results in the CI recipient feeling guilty about any conversation difficulties occurring in the conversation. An aggressive attitude has patients blaming others for their poor speech quality or their inability to meet the needs of the conversation, without these having been expressed.

In this activity a selection of communication settings are outlined and a range of alternative responses is provided. The CI recipient is asked to consider and evaluate the appropriateness of the passive, aggressive and assertive alternative responses for each setting. The exercise offers CI recipients an opportunity: (1) to develop an awareness of the patterns and purposes of assertive communication, (2) to prioritize the listening situations in which they find themselves with regard to expectations for successful communication, and (3) to consider others' willingness and ability to alter the interaction. This exercise (and the one that follows) is particularly suited to a group rehabilitation setting. It offers opportunities for CI recipients to learn from the experiences and responses of other group members, and can be effective in providing models to those CI recipients struggling to address their passive or aggressive conversational behaviours.

Exercise 6: 'Responses to challenging situations'

This exercise offers CI recipients a follow-up to Exercise 5, in which they are asked to create passive, aggressive and assertive responses to four situations.

In doing so, CI recipients have the opportunity further to identify and distinguish passive, aggressive or assertive responses. The purpose of this activity is to begin to develop an understanding of a repertoire of assertive strategies for any given situation. The CI recipient may recognize that many of the 'normal' strategies used in everyday conversational breakdowns are available to them. This can increase the CI recipient's confidence and self-esteem as a communication partner. This activity works well in the group format, often leading to healthy discussion of the different types of communication and their relative value.

Exercise 7: 'Requesting changes in the environment'

This exercise provides a further opportunity to rehearse assertive communication behaviours. It lends itself well to role-play and extended discussion to help develop and reinforce realistic expectations of the resolution of communication difficulties. This exercise contains 10 examples of potential difficulties in everyday conversation settings in which the CI recipient's hearing impairment may require him or her to address potential or actual communication breakdown. CI recipients are asked to complete each item by giving their most assertive response to the situation.

Conversation strategies

Exercise 8: 'Adaptive and maladaptive strategies'

This exercise was developed and adapted from Erdman et al. (1984). People tend to adapt their conversational behaviours to the dictates of the communicative environment. Many CI recipients will report on behaviours in their everyday lives that are dictated by a myriad of communication and lifestyle factors. This exercise introduces the concept of adaptive/ maladaptive communication behaviour and aims to bring under greater conscious control the choice of behaviours that CI recipients exhibit. Given a list of communication strategies, the CI recipient is asked to identify whether he or she feels that a particular strategy or tactic is adaptive (i.e. that it leads to a good, appropriate or useful outcome) or maladaptive (i.e. it leads to an undesirable outcome). The identification of each tactic as adaptive or maladaptive allows discussion about their use and suitability. This exercise can be an effective assessment tool enabling the clinician to identify key areas of difficulty, and is particularly beneficial for early intervention sessions to assist clinician and CI recipient to assess the key aural rehabilitation goals. In a group rehabilitation model the discussion after completion of the exercise offers an excellent opportunity for the CI recipients to discuss and model behaviours that they require from others in the group setting.

Exercise 9: 'Asserting yourself on the telephone'

This exercise outlines a range of common communication difficulties experienced when conversing on the telephone. Six telephone-based conversation difficulties are presented and CI recipients are asked to suggest responses to each by which the conversation difficulty may be addressed. Although telephone conversation has many interactional and social aspects in common with face-to-face communication, the absence of visual speech and speaker cues, the reduced acoustic quality and the lack of speaker identity under certain circumstances make it a difficult situation to deal with for some CI recipients. Allowing the CI recipient to plan and discuss appropriate solution(s) to telephone conversations can be very useful. These strategies may then be used in role-play or trials in the clinic room or as a basis for group discussion.

Tactics for the conversation partner

Exercise 10: 'Effective communication for family and friends'

This exercise is useful when working with both CI recipients and their communication partners. It allows the communication partner to consider some of the tactics that they may implement (e.g. rate of speech or the use of gestures). It offers an opportunity to self-evaluate the communication skills that are important in conversation with adults with hearing impairment. It can be used to foster discussion around expectations of each participant in the communication situation.

Non-verbal communication

Exercise 11: 'Effective communication – non-verbal communication'

In discussion of assertive repair strategies it becomes apparent that some CI recipients have not considered the impact of their own manner and non-verbal messages on communication. This activity provides an opportunity to make CI recipients more aware of elements of non-verbal communication such as facial expression, body language, physical proximity and tone of voice. It aims to raise awareness of these issues and to assess the non-verbal information that these behaviours impart.

Problem-solving

Exercise 12: 'Problem-solving communication difficulties'

This exercise reintroduces work on anticipatory or preparatory strategies, and is based on the commonly occurring characteristics of a particular event or setting. The scenarios, which are more detailed than in earlier exercises, provide CI recipients with opportunities to consider in advance the circumstances in which they might find themselves, and the people, the type of talk and the physical environment that comprise them. This is useful work for CI recipients who may not have well-developed metacommunication awareness or who may be poor at analysing circumstances in which they find themselves communicating regularly. Under careful and structured guidance CI recipients can do this well, even though they have not paid conscious attention to it before.

This exercise presents three scenarios of individuals experiencing communication breakdown as the result of hearing impairment. Although it may be used early on in the programme to assess the CI recipients' awareness of the range of strategies available to them, it is also a valuable exercise at the conclusion of the programme as a summary of the skills learnt. Issues such as use of technology, management of the environment, use of repair strategies, language strategies, assertiveness and relaxation are all pertinent to the examples presented.

Acknowledgements

Much of the background work to the exercises in this chapter was undertaken by the authors and their colleagues at **hear**service (Hearing Education and Aural Rehabilitation service) of the Victorian Deaf Society (now Vicdeaf), in Melbourne, Australia from 1987 until now. The authors wish to acknowledge the rich and exciting environment in which much of this work came into being, and the colleagues and clients who were and continue to be the guidance and inspiration for this work. Some of the exercises set out in this chapter have been taken from the (then) 'Coping with a Hearing Loss' course (now the 'How to Understand Hearing Loss' course) developed and run by the clinical and community education staff at **hear**service. Each exercise taken from the programme is produced under copyright of **hear**service and of the authors and is reprinted with express permission of **hear**service, Vicdeaf. Readers are welcome to reproduce these exercises, and in doing so are requested to include the copyright and reprint information that has been included at the bottom of each page of each exercise. Further enquiries or any comments concerning the exercises or any other work presented here should be directed to one or other of the authors at the addresses at the front of the book.

References

Clark HH, Schaefer EF (1987) Collaborating on contributions to conversation. Language and Cognitive Processes 2: 19–41

Clark HH, Wilkes-Gibbs D (1986) Referring as a collaborative process. Cognition 22: 1–39

Erber NP (1996) Communication Therapy for Adults with Sensory Loss, 2nd edn. Clifton Hill, Melbourne: Clavis

Erber NP (2002) Hearing, Vision, Communication and Older People. Clifton Hill, Melbourne: Clavis

Erber NP, Lind C (1994) Communication therapy: Theory and practice. Research in audiological rehabilitation: Current trends and future directions. Journal of the Academy of Rehabilitative Audiology 27(monograph suppl): 267–87

Erdman SA, Crowley JM, Gillespie GG (1984) Considerations in counseling the hearing impaired. Hearing Instruments 35: 50, 52, 54, 56, 58

Gagné J-P, Tye-Murray NE (1994) Research in audiological rehabilitation: current trends and future directions. Journal of the Academy of Rehabilitative Audiology 27(monograph suppl)

Hetú R (1996) The stigma attached to hearing impairment. Scandinavian Audiology 25(suppl 43): 12–24

Kaplan IL, Bally SJ, Garretson C (1995) Speechreading: A way to improve understanding, 2nd edn. Washington DC: Gallaudet University

Kricos PB, Lesner SA (1995) Hearing Care for the Older Adult: Audiologic rehabilitation. Boston, MA: Butterworth-Heinemann

Lind C (2004) Conversation therapy following cochlear implantation. In: Pedley K, Lind C, Hunt P (eds), Adult Aural Rehabilitation – A guide for CI professionals. Lane Cove, Australia: Cochlear Ltd, in press

Pichora-Fuller MK, Johnson CE, Roodenburg KEJ (1998) The discrepancy between hearing impairment and handicap in the elderly: Balancing transaction and interaction in conversation. Journal of Applied Communication Research 26: 99–119

Trychin S (1988) So That's the Problem! Washington DC: Gallaudet University

Trychin S, Boone M (1987) Communication rules for heard of hearing people. Washington DC: Gallaudet University.

Tye-Murray N (1992) Preparing for communication interactions: The values of anticipatory strategies for adults with hearing impairment. Journal of Speech and Hearing Research 35: 430–5

Tye-Murray N (1994) Communication strategies training. Research in audiological rehabilitation: Current trends and future directions. Journal of the Academy of Rehabilitative Audiology 27(monograph suppl): 193–208

Tye-Murray N (1998) Foundations of Aural Rehabilitation: Children, adults, and their family members. San Diego, CA: Singular.

Tye-Murray N, Schum L (1994) Conversation training for frequent communication partners. Research in audiological rehabilitation: Current trends and future directions. Journal of the Academy of Rehabilitative Audiology 27(monograph suppl): 209–22

Chapter 8
Speech and language therapy in the rehabilitation of an adult with a cochlear implant

SUSAN HAMROUGE AND SARAH WORSFOLD

This chapter has been written as a reference and practical guide for speech and language therapists who would like to have a more specialist knowledge of hearing impairment and its management.

Increasing numbers of speech and language therapists will come into contact with recipients of cochlear implants (CIs) as time goes on because:

- adults continue to be implanted
- the criteria for implantation continue to change
- people are living longer
- implanted children will grow up.

Some CI recipients will have an acquired hearing loss. This could have been sudden or progressive, and the duration of loss at the time of implantation will vary. Others will be congenitally deaf. Hearing experiences and rehabilitation needs will vary within and especially between these groups.

The speech and language therapist may be referred CI recipients in adult clinics in hospitals or the community and, as Stenglehofen (1989) points out, in the context of cleft palate work, speech and language therapists already have a range of relevant skills, i.e.

- interpersonal skills
- observational skills
- skills to elicit speech and language data
- skills to provide a comprehensive assessment of communication
- skills to set goals with the CI recipient (and communicative partners where appropriate)

- skills to design an effective management programme
- skills to carry out remedial procedures
- skills to work in a range of communication modalities.

This chapter aims to look at some of the factors that have particular relevance to the management of CI recipients.

We have found work with adult CI recipients to be very rewarding. CI recipients often take a keen interest in the structure of speech and language. This allows a metalinguistic approach to therapy. Deafened adults may already have worked hard in communicative situations by the time that they arrive in the clinic. Easy communication with someone who is able to take some time with them is much appreciated, and CI recipients are often active in taking responsibility for their own rehabilitation programme. Each person will have had different experiences and will need an individual management programme. This gives plenty of opportunity to learn about new topics that interest the CI recipient and to be creative in devising activities.

The first section of this chapter gives an overview of how deafness can affect both speech perception and production and communication skills. Speech acoustics are reviewed because this information plays in important part in developing a workable management programme.

The section on assessment offers some suggestions that clinicians might find helpful when collecting information on how the CI recipient and his or her communicative partner are coping with communication. Case history information should be gathered from all available sources. The clinician is encouraged to seek information about how well the CI recipient communicates with a variety of people in a variety of situations and locations that are important in his or her everyday life.

The goal-setting section emphasizes the necessity for this to be a joint venture, with CI recipients and their communicative partners both expressing their interests and expectations. The clinician may think that, as a result of assessment, specific communicative goals could be achieved. However, the CI recipient may not wish to spend a lot of time in rehabilitation, and may have relatively limited goals of his or her own. Conversely, CI recipients could have unrealistic expectations, although these should have been tempered by information and counselling given before surgery. In either event, joint goal setting increases the likelihood of success of the subsequent management programme.

The section on therapy and ongoing care offers some practical ideas for rehabilitation. These are taken from what is a limited body of literature and our own experience. Many of the resources (or similar items) will be readily available in speech and language therapy adult clinics, and references for other resources are given.

Finally, case studies are used to illustrate some of the issues that clinicians will face when dealing with this group.

How deafness affects speech

Speech is a complex auditory signal. The auditory components of a speech sound vary in three different parameters:

(1) intensity/loudness
(2) frequency/pitch
(3) timing/duration.

Speech perception

In the cochlea the basilar membrane varies in width and flaccidity along its length and, following the principle of resonance, will respond maximally (i.e. will be maximally displaced) at a specific point along its length when excited by a sound of a specific frequency. Low-frequency tones cause maximum displacement towards the apex, whereas high-frequency tones cause maximum displacement towards the base of the basilar membrane.

Areas along the basilar membrane work as 'filters', because they respond to certain frequencies but not to others. When 'excited', neural fibres in that area start firing in synchrony with the incoming waveform. The frequency that causes maximal displacement in a given area is called the characteristic frequency (CF). The band of frequencies surrounding this frequency to which neural fibres will also respond is called the critical bandwidth (CB). The CB increases with CF so filters responding to low frequencies have narrow bandwidths and 'pass' only a small range of frequencies. Filters responding to high frequencies have wide bandwidths and pass a large range of frequencies. The basilar membrane can be described as functioning as a 'bank of overlapping filters'.

To be able to discriminate speech, three processes operate in the cochlea: frequency resolution, loudness resolution and temporal resolution.

Frequency resolution

Frequency resolution is based in part on the critical band filters described above. These filters are narrow enough in the 500–3000 Hz frequency range to pick out different formants (bands of increased acoustic energy – see below), which contribute to our perception of pitch, intonation, vowel quality and other patterns (e.g. plosion, friction) that cue consonants.

When a person has a sensorineural loss many neural fibres might be non-functional and frequency resolution may be much poorer. However, there is considerable variability between people, so those with similar hearing thresholds may differ widely in their frequency resolution abilities. As filters are broader in the case of hearing loss, in noisy environments more noise will be passed by a filter and will mask the signal being passed in the same filter. This leads to a poorer ability to understand speech in noise. Speech can sound blurred or indistinct and high-frequency components will be difficult to perceive (as a result of very wide filters and upward spread of masking).

Temporal resolution

The ear is very good at decoding small changes in duration. Normally hearing listeners can detect gaps as short as 2–3 ms. As a result of the relationship between filter bandwidth and perception of duration, the ear shows better time resolution at high frequencies. The ability to perceive differences of the order of 10–20 ms is important for the perception of certain sounds, e.g. plosives. The perception of stress and voice-onset timing also depends on this area of processing.

In the impaired cochlea temporal resolution occurs at a rate of 20–30 ms and this can affect the ability to understand speech in noise.

Loudness resolution

Loudness resolution allows perception of the voiced/voiceless contrast, stress and tone of voice (relative intensities of different patterns). Loudness is a subjective term and tones at different frequencies that have the same intensity can be perceived as being of different loudness.

Hearing threshold curves show that the normal ear is most sensitive to tones with frequencies from 100 Hz to 5000 Hz. Sensorineural loss is usually associated with an abnormality of loudness perception called loudness recruitment. Although the hearing threshold is elevated, the rate of growth of loudness with intensity is more rapid than in a normal-hearing ear. A sound can quickly go from being barely audible to being painful for the listener. There are also problems with sound localization.

Formant frequencies

Resonances of the vocal tract are called formants, and their frequencies the formant frequencies. Every configuration of the vocal tract has its own set of formant frequencies. Voiceless sounds have acoustic information across a wide band of frequencies.

Voiced sounds (most obvious with vowels) have narrow bands of increased intensity, which are connected with the particular configuration of the vocal tract for that sound.

The first formant (F_1) is the first band of increased acoustic energy above F_0. As with all formants it can rise and fall independently of higher and lower formants. The next highest band of acoustic energy is the second formant, etc.

Figure 8.1 emphasizes the point that vowel perception is achieved by recognition of the different tongue positions used, producing different formants, which give us different acoustic cues to discriminate between the sounds.

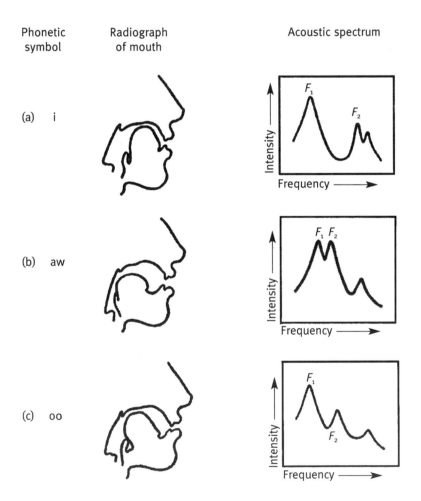

Figure 8.1 Vocal tract configurations and corresponding spectra for three different vowels: (a) i; (b) aw; (c) oo. (Reproduced with permission from Denes and Pinson, 1973, Figure 32, p. 78.)

The formant chart in Figure 8.2 has been adapted from Ling and is a useful reference to have when making decisions about which vowel discrimination tasks need to be tackled.

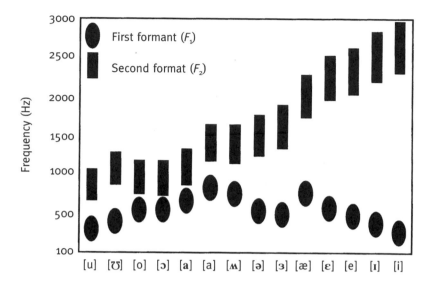

Figure 8.2 Vowel formant chart.

It is also useful to have a visual aid to show people when talking about the relationship of speech sounds to each other, and Appendix 6 is an audiogram of familiar sounds to help you with this.

However, people with similar hearing thresholds may differ widely in their speech perception abilities. This will be more apparent when dealing with people who have received implants after long-term deafness or those born with a hearing loss. Their ability to perceive sounds will have been affected by their degree and type of loss. Consequently, their experience of discriminating sound will be different from those who have suddenly lost their hearing but previously had good perceptual abilities. As a guideline refer to the sample audiograms in Appendix 7. These audiograms will give you some idea what sounds may/may not have been perceived acoustically and therefore the areas of potential difficulty that need reinforcing now that CI recipients have access to a fuller set of acoustic cues. They are only a starting point and other factors, e.g. lip-reading abilities or use of contextual cues, need also to be taken into account.

Below are the features of the speech signal that might be recognized when hearing is available only to the specified level. This information should be useful for planning a hierarchical structure for therapy. Hearing in the speech range up to 250 Hz allows us to perceive the following acoustic features:

- Fundamental frequency F_0
- Non-segmental duration and intensity
- Detect F_1: /u/and/i/
- Voicing cues of some consonants: /k/v/g/
- Detect nasal murmur: /m, n, ng/.

Hearing in the speech range up to 500 Hz allows us to perceive the following acoustic features:

- Detection of the F_1 of most vowels
- Voicing cues in consonants
- Detection of some plosive bursts.

Hearing in the speech range up to 1000 Hz allows us to perceive the following acoustic features:

- F_1 back and central vowels
- Discrimination between /w/ and /j/
- Consonant/vowel (C/V) and V/C transitions
- Discrimination of consonants by manner.

Hearing in the speech range up to 2000 Hz allows us to perceive the following acoustic features:

- Note that this is the key frequency for the perception of speech
- Discrimination of some vowels differing only in F_2 and F_3
- Acoustic information for /l/ and /r/
- May discriminate /w/ and /r/
- Detect more plosive bursts
- Discrimination of affricate bursts
- Discrimination of most vowels based on F_2
- Discrimination of some place cues
- Discrimination of fricative turbulence /h/ sh.

Hearing in the speech range up to 4 kHz allows us to perceive the following acoustic features:

- Discriminates all vowels
- All place cues

- Detection of /s, z/ phonemes:

plurals	copulas
third person	idioms
questions	auxiliaries
possessives	past perfect

Potentially CI thresholds are −20 to 35 dB hearing level (HL) accessed across the speech frequency range. All phonemes are audible in most cases.

Why do we need to know about speech acoustics?

We need to know this because it gives us a baseline for possible speech reception by which to:

- demonstrate the effectiveness of the device
- understand why speech perception errors are made
- plan the content of an intervention programme
- allow hierarchical delivery of tasks.

However, although it is necessary, it is not sufficient information, because other factors are important in speech perception, e.g.

- use and integration of speech-reading information and other non-verbal cues with acoustic information
- signal-to-noise ratio – distractions can be both visual and auditory
- higher-order skills, e.g. learning styles, attention span, etc.
- experience of language – acquired or congenital loss
- age of loss
- sudden or progressive loss.

For any clinician wanting to work in this area, we strongly recommend further reading including *The Speech Chain* (Denes and Pinson, 1993) and similar texts.

How deafness affects speech production

As with speech perception, reviewing the audiogram will give us *some* information about how a CI recipient's speech production may have been affected as a result of reduced ability to monitor his or her own speech output. However, again it is not sufficient information. Well-learnt neurological patterns, anxiety, tiredness and complexity of the message, among other factors, will have an effect on a person's performance.

There is not yet a large body of literature on the effects of deafness on speech production. For overviews of the research the reader is referred to Read (1993), Tobey (1993) and House in Plant and Spens (1995).

It appears that many postlingually deafened adults maintain remarkably normal sounding speech. How this happens, when auditory monitoring has been severely reduced, is not well understood. There may be a link between severity of speech disturbance and the age of onset, as well as the length of time since loss of hearing (Tobey, 1993). Certainly, reduction in speech intelligibility in the context of a congenital loss is often seen.

However, there have been a number of reports of changes in speech production, including nasal resonance and voice control. Articulatory changes are more often seen at the phonetic, rather than the phonological, level. They may have implications for the ability to signal grammatical information, e.g. if /s/ word final is not used, plurals, possessives and third person singular are not indicated.

The following are areas of speech production that have been reported as being vulnerable to change after an acquired hearing loss.

Breath support

Anxiety in the communicative situation, which may be noted on clinic visits, can lead to changes in breath support and control. This can mean that:

- the amount of air available for speech support is limited
- there is an increased use of residual air
- the inspiratory airstream is used for speech
- clavicular rather than diaphragmatic breathing patterns are used
- tension is present throughout the body, dampening easy, fluent movement.

Voice

The quality of the voice relies heavily on auditory feedback. A CI patient's voice may be described as:

- harsh
- breathy
- grating
- pressed.

Problems with timing of voice onset may lead to devoicing or intrusive voicing. Reduction in control of F_0 leads to abnormalities of pitch (level and range). Problems with control of intensity can also occur.

Resonance

As with laryngeal control, control of the soft palate is thought to rely heavily on auditory feedback. Features seen clinically in this population are:

- hyper-, hypo- and mixed nasality
- cul-de-sac resonance/tight pharynx
- reduced differential movement of different parts of the tongue leading to reduced changes in oral resonance.

Phonetics

Segmental aspects are thought to be less often affected than non-segmental aspects of the speech signal. Listed below are features that are most likely to be encountered in both areas.

Segmental

- Cluster reduction
- Changes in vowel length – both reduction and increase
- Generalized backward shift of the vowel space
- Changes in F_1 and F_2
- Omission or substitution of consonants
- Fricative /s/ especially vulnerable.

Non-segmental

- Changes in speaking rate; tendency towards slower rate
- Pauses – too many/too long
- Changes in rhythm
- Uncontrolled or monotonous pitch
- Excess stress and changes in stress patterns
- Tendency towards a limited range of intonation patterns.

How deafness affects communication

The point that emerges is that communicative problems are massively and specially significant for deafened people.

Cowie and Douglas-Cowie (1995)

Deafness affects all areas of life. Even with an implant, and particularly in the early days, it may be difficult to recognize warning signals such as fire alarms and emergency service sirens. Information, such as platform information, public announcements, weather and traffic reports, may be missed and CI recipients may have got out of the habit of going to the theatre or movies for pleasure many years ago. But the information that is really missed by those who have had hearing, and often imperfectly available to those with a congenital loss, is that derived from communication.

Receptive and/or expressive personal communication skills can be affected. Perhaps this would be most obvious in conversation with an unfamiliar speaker, on the phone or talking in a group. Group situations, generally, are difficult and the CI patient's access to clubs, religious and community activities may be significantly affected. Parties are often a source of anxiety rather than enjoyment. Communication difficulties at work can affect a CI recipient's current position, employment prospects and possible chances of promotion.

For communication to be successful in any of these environments, the message must be delivered in a way that the receiver is able to understand. The fluency of communication that we usually expect may be significantly affected, if one of those involved is deaf or severly hearing-impaired. Both or all communicators need to take responsibility for changing their habits as both senders and receivers, in order for communication to remain successful.

Families and friendships can rely heavily on particular habits of communication, e.g. calling from room-to-room rather than waiting to talk until both people are face-to-face. When deafness means that previous habits are no longer successful, changes in relationships may occur. A sudden loss of hearing for one partner can be traumatic for both.

There are a number of ways in which communicative interactions may change when a hearing-impaired person is involved. People with long-term losses tend to have developed coping strategies, which might not help communication, e.g.

- Domination of the conversation, which becomes almost a monologue. This may be to keep control of the situation and not risk misunderstanding because of a change of topic. The listener is forced into a passive role.
- Bypassing conversation by taking action without consulting others.
- Pretending to understand but struggling to work out even the topic of conversation. Hoping that something will be said that will make the subject clear. After 20 minutes of conversation it is very difficult to admit to a stranger that you have understood nothing.
- Blunt question-and-answer conversations using very direct language to avoid the risk of misunderstandings.
- Withdrawing from conversation: limiting offerings to social phrases, or

relying on pen and paper. This affects the dynamics of communication.
- Reliance on family members to become translators, producing a running commentary. Again, this inevitably affects the dynamics of communication.

Communicative partners can also be affected by a need for change in communicative style and:

- withhold information, particularly non-vital information to avoid the need for repetition.
- proceed with a conversation telling the deaf partner that he or she will 'tell them later'. This may or may not happen. In any case it does not allow participation at the time.
- reduce conversation to very simple and limited exchanges, and then quickly make their excuses and leave, to avoid the embarrassment of a breakdown in communication, which they do not feel confident to repair.

Non-verbal aspects of communication can also be affected. This information may be intended, or 'leaked', and be available to others whether or not intended. Frowning while concentrating on understanding or lip-reading may give entirely the wrong impression, without the CI recipient being aware of the effect that this is having. Tiredness can lead to a slumped posture, which gives a 'disinterested' message. Leaning forward to make lip-reading easier may be interpreted as an invasion of another's body space, or an indication of anger, which is not intended.

As communicative situations can provoke a lot of anxiety for those who are deaf, there can be a feeling of isolation and a reduced feeling of well-being. There is much anecdotal evidence of this (Gailey, 2003), and clinically we have often worked with people who feel very inadequate in situations where they fear a breakdown of communication.

For a further discussion of this area see publications by Hogan (2001) and Erber (1988, 1993, 1996, 2002).

Assessment

The aim of assessment is to find out about functional communication – to get a picture of the whole person and his or her communicative relationships. It is necessary to gather information:

- from all available sources
- in a variety of environments.

Listening to the individual, family, friends and work colleagues, where possible, will give information about how communication varies in different situations and with different participants. Both will affect communicative success, and this information is unlikely to be captured simply from formal assessment in a quiet clinic room or audiology booth – even with both communicative partners present. The WHO (2000) classification suggests that assessment covers the following areas:

- Body functions and structures: relevant physiological and psychological body functions and anatomical structures including level of any impairment.
- Activity: the communicative skills of the individual, identifying strengths, needs and difficulties.
- Participation: use of functional skills in communication within the current and likely environments (including different settings, routines and relationships), and the opportunities and need for communicative use in everyday life.
- Contextual factors: the individual's (and partner's where appropriate) perception of the impact of deafness on his or her life. The physical, social and attitudinal environment in which they live.
- Personal factors, e.g. race, gender, educational background and lifestyle.

Considerations before carrying out assessment

Many of the following tips will be familiar to clinicians working with adults who have communication difficulties for a variety of reasons:

1. Implant users may have accompanying problems, e.g. degenerative neurological conditions affecting:
   – communication
   – mobility, which may affect opportunities for communication.
   Clinicians should beware of this. It is easy to attribute all difficulties to deafness, whereas there may be additional language comprehension difficulties and/or memory problems.
2. If the CI recipient's first language has been sign, or the CI patient and/or communicative partner has a different first language from the clinician, it may be necessary to work with an interpreter. Proceed with great caution when using any standardized test with interpreting. A family member could fulfil this role, but this will depend on availability and relationships within the family. Local audiology departments will have contact details for sign interpreters.
3. Be prepared to take time over assessment and allow for (frequent) breaks to reduce the effects of fatigue. Allow pauses for the message to be decoded and language to be processed.

4. Try to arrange for the use of a quiet room, with no interruptions for case history taking. This may not be easy in a busy department where space is at a premium.

5. Be careful about the layout of any room/space used for assessment because this may affect the results obtained. If the clinician sits with his or her back to the window, for example, lip-reading and perception of facial expression are much more difficult than if the face is well lit.

6. Background noise and visual distractions when trying to lip-read can also interfere. For a more detailed description of hearing tactics, see the Oticon entry in Resources at the end of the chapter.

7. Be prepared to use repetition, rephrasing and different modalities during assessment for delivery of both stimuli and responses, especially for explanation of what the CI recipient is expected to do. This will help to ensure that the clinician is testing what he or she intends rather than the fact that instructions have not been understood.

8. If the CI patient has not had good communicative experiences he or she may be reluctant to risk a repeat. The clinician may need to start with areas that are 'safe', and where success is likely, before tackling areas that are perceived as difficult.

9. Encouragement is very important, and it is worth developing a range of appropriate phrases gently to request a further attempt, when there has been a temporary breakdown in communication. If there is a complete failure of understanding, suggest that you try again later. This will take the pressure off and may allow both parties to review what they think was said and try to work out what was meant.

10. Do not pretend that you have understood, because this often becomes obvious when responses are not those expected. Future rehabilitation, which depends on a trusting relationship, will then be compromised.

11. The clinician's body posture (as well as other aspects of non-verbal communication) may be a major source of information, and thought should be given as to what messages are given and received.

12. An unhurried attitude, even when this is not the case, will be an encouragement to the CI recipient. As with other visitors to speech and language therapy clinics, use of direct attention and regular eye contact may facilitate interaction.

13. Watch the listener's reaction to monitor whether he or she is following the message.

14. Speaking in concise complete sentences allows the CI recipient to use his or her knowledge of the rules of language to try to 'fill in' words that he or she has not heard. Similarly, continuing to talk around the same subject will allow better prediction of the kinds of words and phrases that might

be used, and can significantly increase the percentage of the message correctly perceived.

15. Unfamiliar vocabulary such as place names or people's names may cause difficulty and a pen and paper is useful to 'ease' communication along.

Case history

In addition to the usual administrative, medical and biographical information gathered when taking a case history, it is recommended that the clinician specifically consider the following audiological information:

- History of loss (age of onset, congenital or acquired, sudden or progressive, and current hearing thresholds).
- Capability of device used: how many electrodes are inserted? What are the recommended settings?
- Is there consistent use of the implant?
- Are additional devices used, e.g. radio aid, hearing aid in the other ear?
- Access to and use of phone, e.g. minicom, Typetalk, fax and texting.
- Is there tinnitus?
- Are there balance problems?

Communication information

1. Preferred mode of communication
2. Language and modalities (including accents and dialects) used at home, socially and at work
3. Contact numbers if interpreters are used
4. Level of speech-reading skills.

See Appendix 8 for specimen case history form.

Formal assessment and skilled observation

There are very few standardized instruments looking at communication for use with this group, so the results of published assessments should be interpreted with caution. It is suggested that the clinician completes a communication checklist (see Appendix 9), and then probes assessments for areas where there appear to be difficulties. This information can be used to help form the basis of a rehabilitation programme.

Adult CI recipients have a wide variety of history of hearing loss and communicative experience. Consequently, the areas requiring detailed assessment will change with each individual. The following areas are those most often mentioned in the literature and encountered by the authors.

Assessment of the communicative partner's speech, language and communication skills, at least at an observational level, should also be undertaken.

Auditory perception

This refers to the CI recipient's ability to detect, discriminate, identify and comprehend auditory information, both environmental and speech sounds. Audiologists on the implant rehabilitation team may be able to provide some information on test results for speech audiometry.

There is often a discrepancy between the signal delivered by the device and the individual's ability to make full use of that signal, particularly in the early days of rehabilitation. Assessment will give information about a CI patient's functional listening, and may help provide a baseline for an auditory training programme (see Chapters 4-6 for a detailed description of the assessment of auditory perception).

Speech reading

Assessment of this area helps understand how the CI recipient is accessing and synthesizing auditory visual information and the clarity of the communicative partner's lip patterns.

Comprehension of spoken/written/signed language

Unless there are additional medical difficulties, it is not likely that an adult with an acquired hearing loss will have language comprehension difficulties for reasons other than the hearing loss. However, the possibility should be borne in mind, particularly with older people. Good language skills will help understanding by use of contextual cues to fill in information that has been missed at the segmental level.

A congenital loss can be accompanied by limited language skills, and assessment of all modalities should be undertaken. A CI recipient with a congenital loss, or who acquired a hearing loss early in life, may have relied more heavily on the visual channel for language learning. It is important to assess in both the auditory–visual and auditory-alone conditions. Record this information on all assessments carried out, and note any discrepancy with language levels used by the communicative partner. Close collaboration with a sign interpreter should be considered where sign has been used for any significant length of time.

Information from the assessment of language comprehension is important for other members of the interdisciplinary team in their dealings with each CI recipient. It will help decide the choice of their assessments and how instructions are given, in terms of the vocabulary and grammatical complexity used, as well as which modalities are most successful. The information will also affect management decisions and possible provision of a therapy programme. Much auditory training is supported by written material, so reading ability should be noted.

Expressive language

For those with an acquired loss, as with language comprehension, the rules of expressive language are well learnt, and loss of auditory acuity will not affect this knowledge. Expressive language should, however, be assessed if there is a congenital or early acquired loss. It should be noted whether grammatical structures used follow the rules of another (spoken or signed) language, or whether there is free variation. Other items to assess are those that are often unstressed in speech, regularly occur in low-energy positions, e.g. word final, or are more complex grammatically. CI recipients with a long-term hearing loss may fail to indicate some grammatical markers such as plural /s/, as a result of reduced auditory monitoring.

Speech intelligibility

This is often taken to mean how well segmental aspects of speech are produced. However, non-segmental aspects of the speech signal, such as rate of speech, stress placement and rhythm, can significantly affect how much the listener will understand.

It is also true that difficulties at other levels of language will have an effect in this area. Even if speech is not very clear, when full grammatical sentences are produced, the listener is able to use his or her own knowledge of the language to help understanding. Remember that speech intelligibity of both partners is relevant and note factors that cause difficulty in understanding the speech of regular communicative partners.

Phonological repertoire

If the CI patient has an acquired loss, particularly if the loss is recent, use of a checklist may be sufficient to indicate that the phonological system is intact. However, if there is a congenital or perilingual loss a full assessment of their phonological system is advised, because the system may be restricted. An understanding of relationships within the system is necessary in order to devise a rehabilitation programme to improve speech intelligibility. Both segmental and non-segmental features of language should be assessed. The reader is referred to the PETAL assessment (Parker, 1999).

Breath support

The efficiency of breath support for speech should be assessed in all cases. Anxiety and frustration in communicative situations can lead to poor breath support for speech for both the CI recipient and the partner. The following areas should be observed:

- Habitual breathing pattern: clavicular or diaphragmatic
- Breathing pattern for speech: clavicular or diaphragmatic
- Excessive use of residual air for speech
- Breath-holding
- Noisy inhalation
- Speech produced on inspiration
- Control of expiratory phase.

Posture/tension

Assessment of excess tension should be observed in a variety of situations, and with different tasks and communicative partners. The CI recipient and partner may be asked to rank different communicative situations and put them on a ladder ranging from easy to most difficult. This is a technique often used when working with people who stammer, who also experience tension during communication. It gives the clinician a useful insight into the individual's view of him- or herself in his or her own communicative world.

Observation of excess tension in the whole body, head, neck and jaw, and when sitting, standing, walking and talking can be instructive.

Voice

Difficulties with breath support and excess tension can lead to problems with voice control. Again, assessment of both participants in different situations and at different times of the day may lead to varying observations being made (for voice profile see Appendix 10).

It is useful to gather information about how, where and when the CI recipient regularly uses the voice. A judgement can then be made about whether current skills match need. A questionnaire to find out about how general lifestyle might affect voice production can also be helpful (for information on taking care of the voice see Appendix 11). Areas covered might include:

- hydration
- use of alcohol

- smoking
- level of stress
- environmental irritants
- vocal abuse.

Resonance

Assessment of problems with resonance should include evaluation of tension in the head and neck, and an examination of the structure and function of the oral cavity. Note should be taken of the following:

- Hard palate: height, width, scar tissue, fistulae
- Soft palate: length, width, symmetry, uvula, mobility, fistulae
- Palatal competence: blowing, sucking, speech (nasal emission)
- Hypernasality in speech
- Hyponasality in speech
- Mixed nasality in speech
- Tongue: at rest, protrusion, retraction, elevation, depression, lateral movement, differential movement
- Jaw: depression, lateral movement, habitual clenching
- Pharyngeal tightness.

Social and interactional skills

Assessment here should take place in different environments and with a variety of communicative partners. Observations should be made (for all concerned) about interpretation and production of verbal, non-verbal and paralinguistic features, discourse skills, and strategies employed to avoid or repair breakdown of communication. For further discussion of this area see Chapters 6 and 7.

Goal setting

There are four options for management with this group: (1) do nothing; (2) offer advice; (3) indirect therapy; or (4) direct therapy – individual/group.

Each CI recipient and communicative partner will have individual circumstances that might impact on goal setting, including:

- communication skills
- communication needs
- motivation
- other calls on their time
- medical/health status.

The clinician should expect to provide information to the CI recipient and the communicative partner on the nature of the problem and how they propose to tackle it. A major long-term goal is to help the patient gain as much insight as possible. Only then will he or she be able to take responsibility for his or her own rehabilitation and extend the programme outside the clinic.

If goals are to be set and met, clinicians must be aware that, although they bring relevant audiological and linguistic information gathered from assessment, and the skills to provide therapy, what *can* be done may not fit with the CI recipient's (and partner's) aspirations. The clinician will have ideas about which areas will have the biggest effect on communicative performance. However, the patient and partner may choose another skill that they feel is causing them more inconvenience in everyday life, e.g. enjoying music, understanding the TV. Consequently, goal setting *must* be a joint enterprise. This avoids a lot of hard work for no practical gain.

The programme goals should be clear, focused and designed around the CI recipient's goals. Outcomes should be agreed and measurable. Determination that expectations are realistic and goals attainable will also save time and disappointment. There should have been a lot of explanation and counselling before implantation, so it is hoped that this will not often be an area of difficulty.

The therapist and recipient decide together on both long- and short-term goals. It is important too that these should be acceptable to the individual and people in his or her environment. Normal speech may not be appropriate as a goal.

After establishment of a programme, regular reassessment of communication goals is recommended to monitor progress. This helps:

- the CI recipient with self-monitoring
- the clinician with monitoring the programme
- all participants work out what to do next.

Therapy

Considerations before therapy

- Work should include frequent communication partners (FCPs) as often as possible. A friend or relative can be a trusted supporter whose assistance can help the CI recipient become familiar with treatment methods and equipment. However, if he or she has a negative view, it can lead to confrontation, lack of engagement, or domination of sessions and the relationship in general.
- The CI recipient often takes on the burden of responsibility for communication breakdown. If the partner has poor understanding of the

communicative needs, there is little likelihood of significant success. To help overcome this, giving the hearing partner earplugs and asking him or her to follow a series of instructions can give insight.

- The clinician must beware the needs of either partner not being met at the expense of the other. It is not always apparent to hearing partners that they, too, will need to change their communicative behaviour, even though they know that current speech interaction can be frustrating. They are lay people and will need training and support themselves.

- Adopt a pattern of provision that is most likely to lead to success. Timing of any therapy should be agreed, in terms of:

  – number of sessions

  – length of sessions, including breaks

  – when the sessions will be and how they will fit into the rest of the CI recipient's (and partner's) life; many will have work and family commitments and in the period soon after implantation other members of the interdisciplinary team may have meetings scheduled with the CI recipient.

- Some adult CI recipients (particularly older people) may not live with a communicative partner. For those who do, the partner may not be capable of helping or willing to change. Obviously, this will affect how goals are to be achieved.

- Some people will live at some distance from the implant centre or clinic. Regular direct therapy may not be a realistic option. However, filling in a communication diary can be a useful basis for discussion when visits to the clinic are made. Some materials are available for home practice, e.g. 'Hear at Home' programme (Plant, 2002) (available from Med El UK Ltd – see Resources); now that so many homes have video players, it is much easier to make video-tapes and use this medium for home practice. Accompanying detailed written instructions are also advised.

- Any programme will be more successful if the participants are as healthy as possible. It is worth thinking about general lifestyle as part of a rehabilitation programme, and devising a personal action plan (Table 8.1) for areas of concern.

Points made in the assessment section about the clinician's communication style are relevant to therapy too. All of us benefit from the use of clear speech and concise language (see Oticon in 'Resources'). This is particularly true for those with a hearing loss.

- Keep language simple and to the point. Those with a congenital loss or an early acquired loss may need both verbal and written language to be significantly simplified, and it is wise for clinicians regularly to check that they have been understood.

Table 8.1 Personal action plan

Activity	Area of concern	Short-term goal	Long-term goal
Breath support			
General health			
Diet			
Exercise			
Sleep			
Relaxation			
Drugs			
Lifestyle			
Environment			
Support			

- For direct therapy, be prepared to go slowly, progressing with small steps, and to consolidate before moving on. Spend extra time to introduce activities perceived as difficult. Model as much as possible.
- Have written material available during the session and to take home afterwards. If people know that they can refer to this afterwards, they will be happier to concentrate on understanding what is being said during the session.
- Speech work is hard! Use motivating and relevant materials. This will make tasks more enjoyable for all participants and help make skills learnt or practised in the clinic more easily generalized to the outside world – which is, after all, where they are needed. It is worthwhile building up a bank of general interest resources from newspapers, magazines, videos and books. Forms, leaflets, TV listings, phone books and other materials that we need daily are particularly helpful if the CI recipient needs work on language skills, although they can be used profitably with any CI patient.
- Consider presenting materials and information in as many modalities as is helpful in each case. Visual feedback equipment, such as Visi-speech or Laryngograph, although expensive to buy, is very useful if available for use.
- Stenglehofen (1989) suggests that the use of analogies can often be helpful for work with people with a cleft palate. We have found it a useful strategy with the hearing-impaired population.
- Many resources used in other areas of adult communication rehabilitation can be modified for use with CI recipients, but the acoustic

characteristics of materials being used needs to be taken into account when deciding the hierarchy of each activity, going from easy to difficult (see 'Why do we need to know about speech acoustics?').

- Any extra memory load resulting from the need to speech read, as well as to look at written materials and listen, needs to be carefully considered.
- Work on auditory comprehension activities before or concurrently with production work.
- Finally, self-esteem and expectations of success may have been affected by previous unsuccessful attempts at communication. It may, therefore, be worth spending extra time to introduce activities perceived by the CI recipient as difficult.

Hundreds of incidents add up to hundreds of bricks add up to a wall
Abrahams (1972 – in Plant and Spens, 1995)

Posture (Figure 8.3)

Goals

- Reduce unnecessary tension
- Increase understanding and self-monitoring
- Use the body's natural symmetry
- Habituation of relaxed posture.

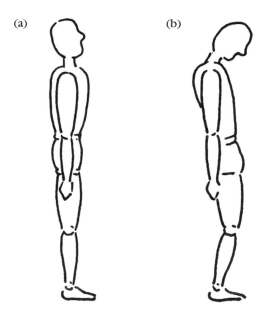

Figure 8.3 (a) Overcorrected and (b) slumped posture. (From Martin and Darnley, 1996, p. 51.)

Describing posture is looking at how we support and balance our bodies against the pull of gravity during daily activities. Small children often have very good control of their posture, but, as we grow up and become subject to increased physical and psychological strains, the body can become subjected to chronic habitual distortions.

Overcorrection of posture should be avoided because this causes tightness. Good posture is important for speech production because it determines the shape and stability of the vessel in which speech sounds are made, and how freely the musculature is able to move.

Caution: watch out for excess tension resulting from concentration.

Exercises

- Lie down with a small paperback supporting the head. Feel the floor/bed supporting weight evenly along the length of the body. Think about the backs of the heels, hips, shoulders and head.
- Sit in a high-backed chair. Feel the chair supporting the weight of the body. There is no need to hold the body upright. The chair should be doing the work. Make sure weight is resting evenly across the pelvis. The head should balance on top of the spinal column. Repeat on an upright chair or stool.
- Stand (in front of a mirror if possible). Have the feet hip-width apart, and make sure the knees are not locked. Balance the weight equally on both legs and make sure that the arms are hanging loosely from the shoulders. Head balanced.
- Stand. Feel as though someone is pulling a string attached to the top of the head. This makes the body feel taller. Feel the distance between the pelvis and the bottom of the ribcage lengthen. This allows more room for movement of the diaphragm. Feel the distance between the collarbone and the lower jaw increase. This allows freedom of movement for the larynx.
- Walking. Make sure the body is balanced equally on either side of the central backbone. Walk tall. Do not lean forwards or backwards. Try to catch an image of your refection in shop windows, etc., to check your posture.

Table 8.2 can be used to record practice of balanced posture.

Many local communities will have adult education classes that address this area, including:

- Alexander technique
- yoga
- swimming
- tai chi
- dance.

Table 8.2 Record of practice of balanced posture

Date												
Lying down												
Sitting												
Standing												
Talking on the phone												
Walking												
Speech reading												
Talking in a group												

Relaxation

Goals

- Reduce excess muscular tension
- Increase kinaesthetic awareness and self-monitoring
- Institute some 'time-out'.

Not everyone will be comfortable with the idea of relaxation, so it is worth taking some time to explain the benefits for speech production. Anxiety in communicative situations can lead to increased tension and practice of these techniques during therapy, when there are no other pressures, can help people become skilled at reducing excess muscular tension when it builds up (Figure 8.4). Audio-cassettes are often suggested for home practice in other rehabilitation programmes. Unfortunately, they are unlikely to be useful with this group. Techniques used in tinnitus are successful, e.g. visualization and imagery may be more appropriate.

Exercises

Repeat each three times:

- Tense arms and fists. Hold for 3 seconds. Concentrate on what this feels like. Let go. Compare this feeling with the feeling of tension. This is the feeling to aim for in communicative situations.

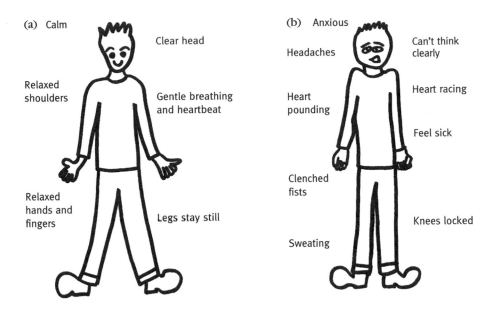

Figure 8.4 Physical and mental feelings: (a) being calm and relaxed versus (b) anxious and tense.

- Tense leg muscles. Hold for 3 seconds. Let go. Compare the feelings of tension and relaxation.
- Tense shoulders. Hold the position. Let go. Compare the feelings of tension and relaxation.
- Tense the whole body. Hold this position. Relax.
- Stretch the whole body. Hold. Relax.
- Screw up the face. Hold. Relax.
- Yawn.
- Chewing keeps the jaw moving and reduces the build-up of tension.
- Stretch lips. Hold. Relax.
- Press lips together. Hold. Relax.
- Lift the back of the tongue and press it against the roof of the mouth. Release.

Use a grid to monitor relaxation practice (Table 8.3).

For further exercises the reader is referred to materials used with other communication rehabilitation programmes, e.g. *The Voice Sourcebook* (Martin and Darnley, 1992) and *Working With Dysarthrics* (Robertson and Thomson, 1986).

Table 8.3 Monitoring relaxation practice

	Week 1	Week 2	Week 3	Week 4	Week 5	Week 6
Relaxed breathing						
Tense arms						
Tense legs						
Tense shoulders						
Tense face						
Five minutes' relaxation						

Breath support

Goals

- Increased understanding and self-monitoring
- Quiet inhalation
- Adequate air supply
- Elimination of shallow breathing
- Controlled exhalation
- Habituation of efficient breathing.

Breathing is a central function, and being asked to perform exercises can make people feel vulnerable. It may be necessary to approach this area gently and explain how good breath support directly affects speech production. Use a simple diagram to explain:

- Breathing to stay alive – inspiration and expiration times are similar.
- Breathing for speech requires quick inhalation and relatively slow, controlled exhalation.
- We speak on the expiration phase.
- We need enough breath to last to the end of an utterance, otherwise we are using residual air, which needs a lot of effort, builds up a lot of tension and is not efficient.

There is also an excellent short video of chest movement during breathing (The Anatomy of the Voice, 1992 – see Organizations/Manufacturers)

> Caution: do NOT encourage excessive effort. This will lead to overflow of tension to other parts of the vocal tract.

Exercises

Watch out for hyperventilation, which can occur with rapid breathing in and out. Go slowly, ask for feedback regularly, and highlight information that the CI recipient gets from kinaesthetic feedback. Sitting or standing in front of a mirror (in the privacy of the home first) can also give useful visual feedback, particularly to stop shoulder movement. Remind about increased tension, and use of the term 'deep' breath rather than 'big ' breath can help.

Establishing diaphragmatic breathing

- Lie flat on the floor. Place hands on the bottom of the ribcage. Feel the ribs move up and down with breathing. Take the hands away and concentrate on the same movement still occurring.
- Stand up. Place the feet hip distance apart. The knees are not locked. With hands on the bottom of the ribs, link fingers loosely across the midline. Feel the fingers pull apart as breath fills the chest, and slide back together on the outward breath.
- Place one hand on the lower ribs and one hand above it, on the upper chest. With an inward breath, only the lower hand should move.
- Place the hands on the waist at the sides. On the inward breath, feel the fingers and thumbs spread, then come back together on the outward breath.

Repeat the above when sitting.

Using the sounds /s, f, sh, th/

- Breathe in for a silent count of two, hold the breath, and breathe out on sssssss for as long as possible. Stop as soon as it becomes effortful.
- Breathe in for a count of two. Hold the breath. Breathe out on sssss as quickly as possible. Compare the feelings when carrying out the first action and this one.
- Using the same pattern of breathing and holding, try the following on sssss:
  - as softly as possible
  - as loudly as possible
  - beginning softly and ending loud
  - beginning loud and ending softly
  - loud–soft–loud
  - soft–loud–soft.

Repeat with /f, sh, th/

Whispering vowel sounds

Produce without 'jerkiness' to the end of a breath:
- ah ee ah ee ah ee
- ee ay ee ay ee
- oo ee oo ee oo
- ee oo ay ee oo ay

Control

Think of these exercises as Morse code. Produce the patterns of sound using /s, f, sh, th/

- —————·—· —————— —·—————— ·—·
- —· —· —————— —· —· —————— — —· —·
- —· —————————— —— —· —· —————————·
- ———————— —————— —· —————————· ——————————
- —· —· —· —· —————————— ·—· —— —·

Pausing

S——————————————S——————————S———————————·
    S———————
Silent count of 2
S——————————————————S———————————————S————
    ———————S
Silent count of 4

Counting in groups

We never take a breath in the middle of a word or in the middle of a phrase. We keep the words together that belong together because of their meaning. This means that we have to make decisions about whether to take another breath when we come to a natural pause (i.e. before each group of numbers in the following exercise). The final number should be as loud and controlled as the first.

1 2 3—————————4 5 6—————————7 8 9———————————
    10 11 12——————
Pause 1
1 2 3—————————4 5 6————————7 8 9——————————————10
    11 12————————
Pause 2
1 2 3 4—————————5 6 7 8——————————9 10 11 12————————
    —·13 14 15 16———————

Pause 3
1 2 3 4 5 ——————————6 7 8 9 10——————————11 12 13
    14 15————————
Pause 4

Count as far as possible on one breath. What does it feel like as you are running out of breath? You should never have this feeling during speech. Stop and take another breath before it becomes an effort.

Voice

Voice use and control are central to the way we communicate in speech. It is part of the way we present ourselves to the rest of the world. If we are confident about the way it sounds, it will be produced at its best. If we are not confident or are feeling tired or insecure for any reason, the voice will be affected. It is thought that auditory monitoring has a big role to play in voice control, and implantation may restore some of this ability. It is, therefore, an area that may benefit from some direct work. For a good quality, well-controlled and flexible voice it is important to have a free and open vocal tract. The reader is advised to revisit the sections above on breathing, posture and relaxation at this point.

Good voice use can be more easily achieved if general health is good. Most of us expect to be able to use the voice without any preparation at all, but if there is pressure on voice production, as a result of reduced monitoring following hearing loss, the vocal tract will benefit from being kept in good order. A hand-out (see Appendix 11) with advice about taking care of the voice can be very helpful – for both CI recipients and their partners.

Voice production

Using line drawings, or if available a rubber model, give a simple explanation of the functions of the larynx in order of importance:

- Stops food and drink entering the lungs
- Helps clear the lungs of infected material
- Fixes the chest for pulling and pushing
- Produces voice.

This is a good starting point for voice work. Most people have never thought about what happens, or have misconceptions. There is also an excellent short videotape of the workings of the larynx (The Anatomy of the Voice, 1992 – see Organizations/Manufacturers) (Figure 8.5).

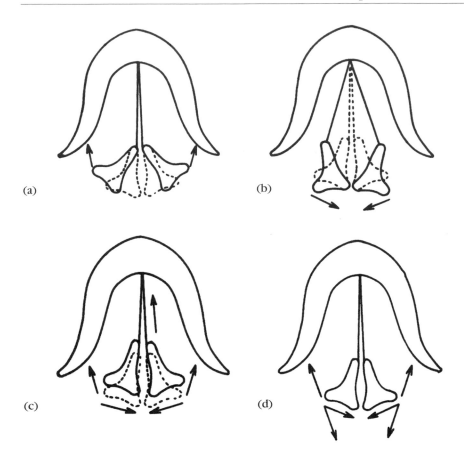

(a)   (b)

(c)   (d)

Figure 8.5 Schematic of the action of some intrinsic laryngeal muscles. (From Zemlin, 1968, p. 174.)

With all exercises, spend time on discrimination as well as production and try to make it fun. People feel highly vulnerable when asked to 'perform' and this increases tension, reducing their chance of success. Take small steps in increasing the difficulty and consolidate at each stage. Having to produce a message as well as control the voice puts a heavy load on monitoring abilities.

Caution: do NOT encourage excess effort.

Voice quality

In general this is not used contrastively in English, but poor voice quality is uncomfortable to listen to, as well as produce, and gives the listener the wrong impression of how the speaker is feeling generally, or about the current topic of conversation in particular. If there is unusual voice quality in addition to restricted phonology, intelligibility can be compromised. Poor voice quality is usually the result of too much or too little effort caused by incorrect tension in part(s) of the vocal tract and/or insufficient breath support.

Review of the sections on posture, relaxation and breath support is advised at this point.

Auditory feedback from an implant may improve the ability to monitor voice quality and encouragement to listen to the sound of the voice in the clinic and at home should be given. Link this with watching for tension in a mirror and monitoring kinaesthetic feedback. If there is any visual feedback equipment, such as Laryngoscope or Visi-speech, available, it will provide valuable information. It takes practice, support and patience for adults with CI systems to synthesize all modes of feedback.

Goals

- Increase understanding and self-monitoring
- Reduce excess tension
- Increase laryngeal control
- Avoid misunderstanding of the speaker's attitude
- Increase intelligibility.

Exercises

- Start with balanced posture.
- Relax
- Use good breath support.
- Practise discrimination of changes of voice quality on single sounds, e.g. /m, ah, oo, ee/. Ask the CI recipient to listen to his or her own and other voices.
- Practise discrimination and production of clear voice quality on words, phrases and longer utterances.
- Use all voiced items first, e.g. *man, name, lane, alone, lion, dine, all alone, more and more, on and on.*
- Watch out for creak as the utterance gets longer, if breath support is limited.
- Use monotone to begin with, then add pitch variation.
- Use written passages read aloud to increase control over a longer utterance.
- Monitor in conversation. Make this a task for recording in a communication diary, so that changes in voice quality at different times of day, as well as different circumstances, can be tracked and discussed at future sessions.

Voice onset

Hard attack can be a result of tension in the vocal tract. It occurs at the beginning of the utterance, particularly on vowel sounds.

Goals

- Achieve relaxed posture
- Good breath support
- Reduced tension around throat
- Increased laryngeal control
- Reduce vocal abuse.

Exercises

- Sit or stand comfortably, with weight balanced and shoulders relaxed.
- Take a gentle deep breath.
- Produce a long /hhhhhh/ sound. With the hand just in front of the mouth, feel the continuous flow of air outwards.
- Add voice to the /hhh/. Use neutral/open simple vowels first, e.g. /hhhhaaahhhh/. Keep the voice on the same pitch.
- Vary the vowel sound used /or, ay, oy, oh, ee/, increasing tension.
- Reduce the length of the initial /h/.
- Produce nonsense words beginning with vowel sounds (e.g. oym, oon, ayb, ohp).
- Produce words beginning with vowel sounds. Watch out for ' habits' of speech creeping back in at this point. Go back to beginning with /h/ if necessary.
- Produce phrases beginning with vowels, e.g.
  - *on the shore*
  - *in the night*
  - *all the way*
  - *and the rest*
  - *if you like.*
- Monitor voice during reading of articles from newspapers or magazines. Use questions requiring answers beginning with vowels, e.g.
  - *Which month comes after July?*
  - *What number comes before 9?*
  - *What is the opposite of odd?*
  - *What is both a colour and a fruit?*
- Monitor use of voice in conversation.

Pitch

A reduction in auditory feedback may have increased reliance on kinaesthetic feedback, and an excessive level of tension throughout the vocal tract becoming habitual. The literature suggests that the fundamental frequency produced by the larynx (F_0) may move towards the expected level following therapy (House in Plant and Spens, 1995).

Goals

- Increase understanding and self-monitoring
- Reduce tension and effort
- Increase laryngeal control
- Carry-over of a suitable habitual pitch.

Optimum pitch and pitch control

Everyone has a pitch that suits his or her anatomy. It is produced easily, without undue effort, and does not need to be pushed. This is the pitch that is produced most efficiently, and much of the speech range is around this note. Men's voices have an average pitch of about 135 Hz, women 235 Hz (Martin and Darnley, 1996) and children 270 Hz (Harris et al., 1997).

Exercises

1. Start with good posture, relax and use good breath support.
2. Hum on a single pitch – one that is roughly the same as the cough/laugh.
3. mmmmmmmmmmmmmmmmmmmmmmmmmmmmmmm. Feel the vibration on the throat by placing the fingertips on the Adam's apple.
4. Repeat a hum, maintaining the same pitch mmm——-mmm——- mmm——mmm.
5. Repeat (3) and (4) using vowel sounds, e.g. /ah, or, ee/.
6. Hum on a single pitch in the lower half of the voice. Use the fingertips to feel the vibration on the breastbone.
7. Hum on a single pitch in the upper half of the voice. Feel the vibration on the nose.
8. Glide down the scale on a hum.
9. Glide up the scale on a hum.
10. Repeat (8) and (9) on vowel sounds.
11. Glide from mid-range to a high note on a hum.
12. Glide from mid-range to low on a hum.
13. Repeat (11) and (12) on vowels.

14. Glide high—-low—-high.
15. Glide low——high——low.
16. Repeat (8), (9), (11), (12), (14) and (15) on words, e.g. *no, yes, really.*
17. Practise phrases and sentences with rise and fall of pitch, e.g. 'It's raining, we're happy, go home, no time'. Encourage reflection. A new sound and feel to the voice takes some getting used to!
18. Practise use of tag questions, e.g. 'Isn't it?', 'Can't we?', 'Don't you?'
19. Use mock arguments, e.g. 'You are late', 'I'm not', 'You are', 'No, I'm not', 'Yes, you are', etc.
20. Practise with friends and family. They will need to get used to the new pitch too.

For more exercises and detailed discussion of voice work the reader is referred to the traditional texts, which will be readily available in voice clinics. Other useful resources are books of audition pieces, monologues and duologue or double-hander plays.

Volume

This is an area that often causes embarrassment for the CI recipient, family and friends. The voice needs to carry to an intended audience but should not be so loud that it makes them uncomfortable. The use of a cheap sound level meter can give useful visual information to match with visual and auditory feedback (see Organizations/Manufacturers). See Appendix 6 for an audiogram of familiar sounds. This can be used as a starting point for discussion about the range of loudness of sound.

Goals

• Increase understanding and self-monitoring
• Match volume to the environment
• Reduce use of excess volume.

Exercises

• Use a sound level meter to register a variety of environmental sounds including speech. This gives a framework into which CI recipients can fit their own voice.
• Divide a range of environmental sounds into loud and quiet. This makes sure that everyone's perception of these labels is understood and, if they differ, it can be addressed and a compromise reached.
• Use more air to increase volume and not effort (refer back to breathing exercises).

- Practise giving vowel sounds full weight as these carry the volume of speech.
- Practise reading at approximately 60 dB.
- Practise reading at approximately 40 dB.
- Practise a short reading at 80 dB+.
- Compare feedback in all available modalities.
- Add varying degrees of background noise (radio or audio-cassette) and try to match an appropriate voice level.
- Agree non-verbal signals, which will allow a hearing partner to indicate the presence of background noise in unfamiliar places.
- Agree non-verbal signals, which allow the hearing partner to indicate that an increase or decrease in volume is required.
- If there is a need to speak to large audiences, e.g. for work or a bride's father's speech, think about the use of amplification to avoid pushing the voice and increasing tension. Get used to a venue before having to 'perform'. Warm up the voice first.

Resonance

This is another area that is thought to rely heavily on auditory feedback for monitoring, so after implantation it may respond to therapy. Good resonance allows the voice to project without increased effort. If the laryngeal note is poor, however, good resonance can help only to a limited extent.

> Caution: do NOT encourage excess effort.

Goals

- Increase understanding and self-monitoring
- Reduce excess tension
- Allow vocal note to be projected.

A simple line drawing of the cross-section of the vocal tract will help in discussion of resonance, and the role of the chest, throat and skull (including how the nasal cavity and sinuses can be coupled and uncoupled to the rest of the vocal tract) should be pointed out. Nasal sounds have relatively high acoustic energy, so they should be some of the easiest to detect.

Exercises

1. Place fingertips on the top of the breastbone. Feel the vibration when humming on a low note.
2. Place the fingertips on the nose. Feel the vibrations when humming on a high note.

3. Place the fingertips on the nose and feel the vibration differences for /m/ and /b/, /n/ and /d/, /ng/ and /g/.
4. Place the fingers on the nose and chest as above. Feel the strength of vibration move from one position to the other when humming up and down the scale.
5. Place the fingertips on the top of the head. If there is good resonance it will be possible to feel vibration here.
6. With open mouth, breathe in quickly in a gasp, as though surprised or shocked. Feel the cold rush of air in the throat. Try to maintain this open position and say a vowel sound /ah/.
7. Place the lips gently together and hum. The lip closure is the first barrier to the escaping airstream. If the throat is 'open' and relaxed, it is possible to get a tickle on the lips.
8. With fingers positioned as in (3) above, try some sentences with big intonation changes, e.g. 'Are you really!', 'I certainly am not!!!!!', 'Well, I never!'

Caution: do NOT encourage excess effort.

Phonetics and phonology

Goals

- Increase understanding and self-monitoring
- Increase intelligibility, not necessarily to give beautiful speech
- Consider expanding the phonological system at segmental and suprasegmental levels to allow differences to be signalled
- Stop partners over-articulating
- Check assessment results for articulation difficulties and compensate where possible if the CI recipient is keen.

Caution: do NOT encourage excess effort.

For some CI recipients speech monitoring may take a great effort and it may be possible to maintain 'my best speech' only for short periods, e.g. for interviews, speeches. Less intelligible speech may be the norm and be quite adequate with family and friends.

Work on speech perception should be undertaken before, or concurrent with, production, to establish the relationship between perception and production for self-monitoring (see also Chapters 4-6 on auditory training).

Clinicians must consider the acoustic characteristics of speech to indicate the sequence of introduction. The following list shows which aspects of phonology are easier and which are more difficult when working on duration, intensity and frequency (item 1 is the easiest).

Segmental

Duration
1. Consonant manner – phoneme duration
2. Consonant voicing
3. Vowels/diphthongs

Intensity
1. Vowels – open vs closed
2. Consonants – plosives vs nasals – loud to soft fricatives

Frequency
1. Differing F_1 tongue height
2. Differing in F_2 tongue height
3. Consonants differing in place

Non-segmental

Duration
1. Short/long
2. Long/interrupted
3. Fast/slow
4. Words varying in number of syllables
5. Sentences varying in number of syllables

Intensity
1. Loud/medium/soft vocalization
2. Stress patterns in words
3. Stress patterns in sentences

Frequency
1. High/mid/low vocalization
2. Male vs female identification
3. Questions vs statements

Work on the following areas is most likely to have a positive effect on intelligibility:

- Rate of speech: use an alphabet board to spell the first letter of each word while speaking to help slow down and increase intelligibility.
- Syllables: use exercises such as practice recognizing the correct number used in words, phrases and sentences
- Stress placement: use exercises such as unstressed first syllables (varies

with accent) to show verb/object, e.g. obJECT versus OBject, to indicate new information, e.g. 'it was a **blue** carpet' versus 'It was a blue **carpet**'.

Language comprehension

It is unlikely that someone with a hearing loss acquired as an adult will have difficulties with comprehension, unless it was a result of, for example, head injury, or there is a co-occurring neurological problem such as stroke. CI recipients with a congenital hearing loss may, however, have such difficulties, and full assessment will reveal areas of difficulty on which to base a management programme. The content should be functional, rather than based on a developmental model, and use relevant everyday materials.

As people age, hearing perception, vision and working memory reduce and thus the ability to integrate information from different modalities is also reduced. This will not affect all elderly CI recipients but it is worth bearing in mind when considering therapy with this group.

After implantation, some aspects of grammar that were previously not detectable, e.g. word-final markers, unstressed elements in connected speech (auxiliary verbs, pronouns and prepositions), may now be heard, and it may be possible to include them in therapy.

In all tasks, consider not only the linguistic complexity, but also the acoustic characteristics of the material used, so that it can be presented hierarchically. Lack of success may be the result of difficulty with auditory discrimination, rather than the grammatical content.

Expressive language

CI recipients with an acquired hearing loss are unlikely to have difficulties in this area, although reduction in auditory monitoring skills can lead to omissions and deletions in connected speech. Those with a congenital or early acquired loss will need a full assessment on which to base a management programme, if the patient is keen to develop his or her skills.

As above, consider the acoustic difficulty of material chosen and present hierarchically.

Interactional skills

Clinicians will be used to the idea of working in groups to develop skills in this area. Other group members:

- act as auxiliary counsellors
- provide real-life models
- share experiences and empathy
- take pressure off the individual.

In our experience, to reduce anxiety it is essential to have a structure to the group that is clear to all participants. This includes giving an overview at the beginning and a timetable for each session.

On a practical level it is helpful to have a set of numbered cards, which are turned over to match the task or item in the list that is currently being addressed. All group members can then be prepared, will be more able to predict and are more likely to succeed.

For a more detailed discussion of this area see Chapter 7.

Case examples

These three case examples are used to illustrate the different ways a speech and language therapist can be involved with a CI user.

Case 1

Sally had moderate learning difficulties. She had a diagnosed sensorineural hearing loss from the age of 5 years but derived benefit from hearing aid usage and was a consistent hearing aid wearer. Her speech and language had developed well with good speech intelligibility and mature sentence structure. When Sally was 17 years old her hearing began to deteriorate and by the time she was referred to the CI programme she was not able to access speech sounds via hearing aids. Sally lost all her self-confidence and became increasingly withdrawn. The CI team could not get her to perform on the standardized speech perception assessments to assess suitability for a CI and she was reluctant to communicate in general.

The speech and language therapist developed a resource of picture material to assess whether Sally's expectations were appropriate for the implant. The material also assessed speech perception skills in a non-threatening way and the go ahead was given for surgery. The quality of life for Sally changed tremendously and she is now able to follow speech without lip-reading. She still does not comply with the requirements of the standardized assessments. The speech and language therapist was able to adapt materials for assessment and teach Sally the tasks required after switch-on to facilitate optimum use of the speech processor.

Case 2

Dennis was a relatively young man of 45 when he became deafened through acute illness. He was not a good lip-reader and his speech was largely unintelligible. There was concern that he had cognitive difficulties after his illness. The speech and language therapist worked with him on a weekly basis pre-implant to establish whether there were any language-processing difficulties. This did not seem to be the case, so the decision was made to offer him a CI. His quality of life also improved tremendously. He had poor breathing patterns and as a result little control over his rate of expiration. Before implantation a lot of work was carried out on breath control using the same approach as for the dysarthric population with the aid of visual resources. With the newly introduced auditory feedback loop, he was able to exert some self-control over his voice intensity and knew how to control it, although breath control remained a significant problem. In addition, he thought that communication breakdown was always someone else's problem although he developed strategies and became more aware of his communication partner's needs.

Case 3

Jane received a CI system when she was 37 years old. Spoken English was not her first language but it was intelligible. Jane could use sign language fluently and was an excellent communicator. The most obvious feature of Jane's voice was her falsetto voice quality. The implant team felt that this needed modification now that she had access to audition but Jane and her family were happy with her voice – it was part of her identity and so the speech and language therapist did not offer intervention.

Resources

Aronson A (1990) Clinical Voice Disorders. New York: Thième
Boone D (1977) The Voice and Voice Therapy. London: Prentice Hall
Bradford B (1988) Intonation in Context. Cambridge: Cambridge University Press
Gallaudet College (1985) Structured Tasks for English Practice. Washington, DC: Kendall Green Publications, Washington Resource
Korky P, Thomas V (1987) Winnie the Witch. Oxford: Oxford University Press
Maisel E (1979) The Alexander Technique. London: Thames & Hudson
Martin S (1987) Working with Dysphonics. Oxon: Speechmark
Martin S, Darnley L (1992) The Voice Sourcebook. Oxon: Speechmark
Med El UK Ltd, Bridge Mills, Huddersfield Road, Holmforth, W. Yorkshire HD9 3TW
Oliver M, Sweeten S (1996) You Should See My Cat. London: Scholastic Children's Books
Oticon. Clear Speech. Oticon, PO Box 20, Cadzow Industrial Estate, Hamilton, Lanarkshire ML3 7QE
Robertson S, Thomson F (1986) Working with Dysarthrics. Oxon: Speechmark
Robertson S, Tanner B, Young F (1989) Dysarthria Sourcebook. Oxon: Speechmark
Stenglehofen J (1989) Working with Cleft Palate. Oxon: Speechmark
Stephens D, Gianopoulos I, Kerr P (2001) Determination and classification of the problems experienced by hearing-impaired elderly people. Audiology 40: 294–300

Organizations/Manufacturers

Link – The British Centre for Deafened People, Eastbourne, E. Sussex. Tel: + 44 1323 638230

Voice Care Network UK, 29 Southbank Road, Kenilworth, Warks CV8 1LA. Tel: + 44 1926 864000; email: vcnuk@btconnect.com; website: voicecare.org.uk

Video: The Anatomy of the Voice (1992). Michael Howes Productions, 6 Theed Street, Waterloo, London SE1 8ST

Laryngograph Ltd, 1 Foundry Mews, London NW1 2PF

Sound Level Meter Model 8928 A2, Instrument Corp. Website: www.a2-instrument.com.tw £49.99

Visi-speech, Millgrant Wells Ltd, 7 Stanley Road, Rugby CV21 3UF

References

Cowie R, Douglas E (1995) Speakers and hearers are people: reflections on speech deterioration as a consequence of acquired deafness. In: Plant G, Spens K-E (eds), Profound Deafness and Speech Communication. London: Whurr Publishers: pp. 510–27

Denes P, Pinson E (1973) The Speech Chain: The physics and biology of spoken language. New York: Bell Laboratories, Anchor Books

Denes P, Pinson E (1993) The Speech Chain. New York: Freeman & Co.

Doyle J (1998) Practical Audiology for Speech-Language Therapists. London: Whurr

Erber NP (1988) Communication Therapy for Hearing Impaired Adults. Abbotsford: Clavis

Erber N (1993) Communication and Adult Hearing Loss. Clifton Hill, Melbourne: Clavis

Erber NP (1996) Communication Therapy for Adults with Sensory Loss, 2nd edn. Clifton Hill, Melbourne: Clavis

Erber NP (2002) Hearing, Vision, Communication, and Older People. Clifton Hill, Melbourne: Clavis

Gailey L (2003) Psychosocial Rehabilitation: The LINK perspective. Paper presented at the 2nd International Adult Auditory Rehabilitation Conference, Portland, Maine, USA May 2003

Harris T, Harris S, Rubin J, Howard DM (1997) The Voice Clinic Handbook. London: Whurr

Hogan A (2001) Hearing Rehabilitation for Deafened Adults – A psychosocial approach. London: Whurr

Martin S, Darnley L (1992) The Voice Sourcebook. Oxon: Speechmark

Martin S, Darnley L (1996) The Teaching Voice. London: Whurr

Maxim J, Bryan K (1994) Language of the Elderly. London: Whurr

Parker A (1999) PETAL. Oxon: Speechmark

Plant G, Spens K-E (1995) Profound Deafness and Speech Communication. London: Whurr Publishers

Plant G (2002) Hear at Home: A home training program. Innsbruck, Austria: MED-EL.

Read T (1993) Speech production in postlingually deafened cochlear implant users. In: Cooper H (ed.), Practical Aspects of Audiology Cochlear Implants: a practical guide. London: Whurr

Robertson S, Thomson F (1986) Working with Dysarthrics. Oxon: Speechmark

Stenglehofen J (1989) Working with Cleft Palate. Oxon: Speechmark
Tobey EA (1993) Speech production. In: Tyler R (ed.), Cochlear Implants: Audiological foundations. San Diego, CA: Singular Publishing Group
WHO (2002) International Classification of Diseases and Related Health Problems. 10th revision. Instruction Manual Volume 2.
Zemlin WR (1968) Speech and Hearing Science. London: Prentice Hall

Chapter 9
Integrating psychosocial aspects of rehabilitation in your programme

ANTHONY HOGAN WITH ANDREA LYNCH

The viewpoint offered in this book is that a planned and well-structured process of rehabilitation, supported by clear programme aims and objectives, will greatly enhance the quality and efficiency of the services that we can offer to deafened adults. Central to this perspective is that the clinician has a heuristic (a mind map) of what he or she is doing with the cochlear implant (CI) recipient and how the process of rehabilitating the recipient occurs overall. In this chapter we extend the work of structuring your intervention by looking at how you go about addressing the psychosocial needs of your CI recipients. It is our view that a consideration of their psychosocial needs is central, not marginal, to aural rehabilitation. People present for assistance at your clinic because deafness has disrupted their lives and they wish to do something about this disruption with a view to moving on.

It can be seen from Figure 9.1 that the intervention has a clear beginning, middle and end. The programme starts with a process concerned with engaging the client in a helping relationship. The strategies for doing this have been documented elsewhere (Hogan, 2001). In this chapter, we want to develop these ideas by looking at them in greater detail. The entire implant intervention is a helping relationship wherein the therapist is having to work with, motivate, console, placate, temper and otherwise enable the CI recipient to manage the vast array of emotions, frustrations and challenges that are endured during this process of remaking him- or herself as a hearing person. It is to the process of managing this task that we now turn.

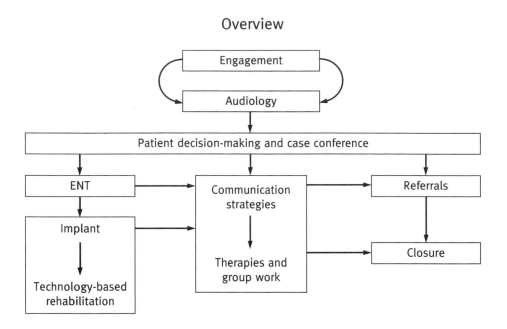

Figure 9.1 An overview of the implant rehabilitation process (Hogan, 2001).

Engaging the CI recipient

A unique set of circumstances surround deafened adults when they present for assistance at a CI clinic. The onset of deafness has very much disrupted the trajectory of their lives. Via the media, people learn that the CI is a miraculous technology that *cures* deafness, and that this device can be obtained from a CI clinic where a team of happy professionals awaits to transform the next lucky person's life into something better.

On the face of it, this appears to be a winning scenario: an excellent technology, competent surgeons, patients in need, and willing and able clinicians. The experienced clinician knows that this process is complicated. First, we cannot guarantee the outcome with the device. Second, we cannot guarantee how any one patient will work with the device. The technology is the technology and no doubt it will continue to improve, but in the meantime we have to make the most of what is available. What we can do a lot about is how we work with patients to ensure that they get the very best they can out of the device as it stands today. The purpose of this chapter is to highlight possible pitfalls in the process of engaging and sustaining the CI recipient in a helping relationship and to suggest strategies for managing the inevitable difficulties that will arise. In Chapters 4–8 and 10, strategies for structuring your rehabilitation programme have been addressed (see also Hogan, 2001). These materials described strategies for setting up your overall programme with regard to psychosocial issues, initial counselling and psychosocial assessment strategies that may be used by you and, in particular, the psychologist or counsellor on your team. These principles are briefly revised here.

Recognizing where your CI recipient is coming from

People are complex and no two individuals are the same. Although it may be obvious that a CI recipient is deaf and that a CI will assist their deafness, this is not a sufficient reason to offer them one. Although the person's physiology may be ready for implantation, it should not be assumed that the rest of him or her is ready. Just as a person, for example, with unmanaged high blood pressure may need a specific programme of assessment and treatment before surgery, so we must look at the psychosocial support needs of the CI recipient before proceeding with the intervention as well. Psychosocial issues are not so much barriers to successful implantation as barriers to good clinician–patient interaction and an optimal outcome from the use of the device in each instance.

First, let us stand back for a moment and reflect on the research about CI recipients' needs and aspirations. Comparing deafened adults as a group with the rest of the community, we find a number of things: they have poorer health; if of working age, deafened people have a greater likelihood of being under-employed or unemployed (perhaps having retired early as a result of their disability), they live on low incomes and many have had their educational outcomes adversely affected by the progressive yet early onset of their hearing loss. Many experience reduced self-confidence. Further, in the wider community, there are notions that people with hearing loss tend to be suspicious or even a little paranoid. Although there is little hard evidence in the research literature to support this negative view of our CI patients, it is a reality that they have to deal with frequently. At a personal level these clients have very real goals for the outcomes of their rehabilitation experiences. They may wish to be able to converse with significant family members such as a spouse, children or grandchildren. They may have things that they wish to do with their life, opportunities to pursue. Many simply want to be able to feel more confident in themselves and more secure in their work. For others, issues of safety and environmental awareness are the primary motivators. Single people may be seeking a relationship or simply wish to extend their circle of friends. People in relationships might have things about the relationship that they hope hearing will change, like the story of Rick, discussed in Chapter 1.

It is the accumulation of these life events, experiences, disappointments, successes and ambitions that psychologically oriented clinicians may often refer to as the CI recipient's baggage. We all have baggage; in fact we all live with the psychological accumulation of our own life events. Often the factor that separates people seeking counselling help from those who do not is simply the sequence of events that occur in life, such as timing and the proximity of events. In addition to their deafness, these CI recipients have had to manage a whole series of difficult life events that most people would call stressors. Some of these factors are on-going insecurity in employment, adverse health events as well as constantly managing a stigmatized identity. In bringing a person into an implant programme it is important to gain an insight into their baggage, not for the sake of it, but to identify factors that may adversely impact on the progress of the CI recipient through the programme. Specific recent life stressors such as the death of a close friend or family member, loss of a job, change of house, marriage or divorce, birth of a child, etc. are factors of concern. In deciding to pursue an implant sooner rather than later, the patient's overall resilience needs to be considered. This is one situation where the input of the counsellor is important. The question, once again, is not so much about the suitability of the individual for implantation, but about the timing. Realistically, except in the case of postmeningitic conditions, or someone with a rapidly progressive hearing loss, most adult implantations do not have a great urgency factor attached to them. So, it is not unreasonable to allow a few months of psychological healing to take place in order to ensure that the person has his or her best chance of maximizing the benefit of the interventions offered. Alternatively, if implantation *has* to proceed for some reason of urgency, additional support and resources may need to be put in place for such a CI recipient because it is likely that he or she will have higher support needs down the line. As the adage goes, fail to plan, plan to fail. What tends to occur presently is that such individuals persistently present post CI with a range of technology-related difficulties, such as the ever-imperfect map. Clinicians spend a lot of time re-mapping processors and trying to re-motivate the CI recipient, when their concerns are in fact of a psychological or support nature and would be better addressed as such.

The second point of focus with regard to engaging clients is that people often have complex motives for seeking out assistance. Specific individuals are not always conscious of these motives and a direct question will not always draw such motives out. Rather, interviewing these individuals about their lives, experiences, difficulties and concerns needs to be pursued and coupled with skilful questioning and counselling, before such issues become apparent. Usually we use open-ended rather than closed questions such as

'Would you mind taking a few moments to tell me about what happened to your hearing?'

You may recall the detail of Rick (in Chapter 1). Rick was a man who really wanted a CI to make up to his wife for supporting his deafness for so many years. An implant, in the first instance, was never going to deal with the issues of guilt, inadequacy and indebtedness that he felt towards his wife. Had this man undergone systematic counselling before pursuing an implant, he may have accepted his outcome and made the most of it. Of course he did not accept the outcome because the feelings of guilt and so on were still present after the intervention. Such feelings can be so omnipresent that they overshadow the real gains that a CI recipient might make as a result of the intervention. Factors such as these may be seen as barriers to a good outcome rather than barriers to proceeding with implantation. Central to understanding and addressing the needs of a CI recipient in a comprehensive way is to think about the aims of your programme. If the aim of the intervention is simply to implant the person in a procedural fashion and the sole focus of the intervention is to establish a stimulation of the auditory nerve, little or no regard has to be paid to the broader psychosocial issues of concern to the CI recipient. In reality, however, implant clinics are about enabling people to get on with their lives, to take their part in the world, as Alexander Graham Bell put it. Programmes as such do not take such a narrow focus. This is not to say that establishing usable auditory input is not an important objective within an intervention, but rather that this goal is one of a series of goals that needs to be addressed.

At times clinicians are aware that a specific person has difficulties or they find that the CI recipient will not comply with reasonable requests to undertake pre-implant rehabilitation. When asked why they persist with such individuals, these clinicians have said that, if they persisted with their concerns or refused to implant the person until such concerns were addressed, the client would go to another programme and that basically they needed the business. You do not need this CI recipient with his or her current disposition, and in fact if you do proceed, he or she will cost you so much time that it will not be worth the business at all, yet alone the stress that you will get. If individuals are not motivated to comply with reasonable clinical requirements before implantation, when motivation to get what they seek (i.e. the implant) is at its highest, they certainly will not be motivated to comply post-implant when they have what they perceive to be a 'lousy' result or they find that they must now comply with rehabilitation directives in order to gain benefit from the device. It is natural for a clinician to want to help individuals and to try to get them the best outcome. However, it has to be accepted that some clients will use our own best nature against us, and work this good intent to their own advantage. In such circumstances things are not likely to go well and it may be better for all concerned to let the person go until he or she is 'ready' to conform to the requirements of a quality intervention.

In summary, there are a range of CI recipient needs that can be identified in the initial stages of intervention. If such issues are not identified or left unaddressed at this time, particularly those that will impact on the individual's longer-term motivation to persist with the device, problems will follow. These problems will involve you in extended efforts later on to fix that which was always broken. Unfortunately, the CI recipient will now blame the problems on you and the intervention, rather than readily addressing his or her own problems and needs. As well, you will have put in a lot of time, effort and resources into what may well become a poor outcome.

Expectations

When individuals present for an implant, they are implicitly looking for a solution to their deafness. At the psychological level, they are looking at a strategy that will enable them to continue on with living their life as close to normal as possible. In these instances, normal refers to 'life as it was before I was deaf'. For many this aspiration is unreal; for others the extent to which this goal can be achieved will be realized only after the procedure and rehabilitation are complete. Certainly, by 6 months after switch-on, everyone will have a very good idea as to the overall result of the intervention. As outcomes are in fact indeterminable before the intervention, the expectations of the CI recipient need to be managed. It greatly aids this process to work with clients to identify what they hope to get out of the rehabilitation programme and to distinguish between results that may be achieved by the device and outcomes that will have to be achieved through auditory or communication training. The Code–Muller Protocols (Code and Muller, 1992; Hogan and Code, 2001) provide a useful counselling strategy for enabling clients to articulate their hopes and aspirations. Coupled with artful questioning, the counsellor or skilled clinician will be able to assist the CI recipient to identify expectations and also to temper such expectations with regard to the results that the device might achieve and the things that will need to be worked on in auditory and communication training sessions. For a detailed discussion on pre-implant expectation counselling the reader is referred to Chapter 2.

At some point in time (typically around 3 months after switch-on), the CI recipient becomes aware of the limitations of the device. It becomes clear that no further optimization of the psychophysical parameters is possible. In some listening environments, communication remains difficult even with the use of assistive listening devices. A client may also realize that other hoped-for changes to his or her life have not occurred. The client is now ready for a more holistic problem-solving approach to the remaining communication problems. One approach to communication therapy is described in Chapter 7.

Deafened people often struggle to obtain or retain their employment. Each person's situation will be different and needs to be approached as such. Some are in employment but are struggling to cope and/or have been unable to gain promotions. Some, for example, have had to leave a previous job as a result of communication difficulties and are unsure what type of work they should be aiming to obtain. Communication is not always the reason why some individuals have become unemployed, so the precipitating factors need to be clarified. Either way, with reduced confidence and reduced communication abilities, individuals may find it very difficult to obtain a new position.

Vocational rehabilitation aims to assist an individual to obtain or retain employment. For many people work is very important, not only to meet financial needs but also to retain self-worth and good health. It is important therefore to ensure that your CI recipients have access to appropriate levels of vocational support.

Vocational rehabilitation providers can:

- assess a person's skills and abilities, preferences/goals and limitations in relation to employment
- identify barriers to obtaining or retaining employment
- design and provide interventions that reduce or overcome these barriers including:
  - adjustment counselling and development of disability management strategies
  - vocational assessments and counselling to identify work/career options and training needs
  - information and access to suitable training (courses or on-the-job training)
  - training and support in job search
  - post-placement support, including support to obtain 'reasonable accommodation', education of co-workers and advice/provision of workplace aids.

The CI clinic generally provides what is considered secondary (second stage) rehabilitation, which is aimed at restoring maximum auditory function in order to reduce communication disability. Vocational rehabilitation providers such as CRS Australia focus on tertiary (third-stage) rehabilitation, which aims to reduce the barriers to full social participation associated with disability by maximizing a person's capacity to participate in the workforce. This is achieved through a range of interventions aimed at reducing the impact of disability, e.g. by enhancing the person's abilities, but also at bringing about change in the workplace environment. A well-known strategy for enhancing the work environment is the education of employers and co-workers about deafness and appropriate communication strategies. Of course, many workplaces may say that they have 'done' such training. It would be a rare workplace that could complete a one-off in-service training programme and in turn implement and maintain an auditorially sustainable environment. Staff change, work settings are rearranged and new work practices are constantly being introduced. Refresher programmes, preceded by a communications audit, should be offered to such workplaces on a routine basis and the schedule for such interventions determined in conjunction with the human resources department of the site concerned. As a guide, training offered every other year may be seen as a minimum level of follow-up to a workplace with well-established communication protocols.

Referral to a vocational rehabilitation agency would follow implantation and would be timed for when the CI recipient's auditory functioning has stabilized, the most intensive period of auditory rehabilitation is completed, and he or she is psychologically ready to focus on an employment goal. In reality, as a result of implant clinic waiting lists and the lengthy assessment processes, clients may be referred pre-implant.

It is essential that the implant clinic and vocational rehabilitation agency communicate about the best timing of a referral for an individual. The potential complexities surrounding a given client (e.g. poor health, stress, anxiety and depression, financial pressures and marital/relationship difficulties) need to be taken into account and addressed in a systematic way. The implant clinic and vocational rehabilitation agency can work together to ensure that these issues are addressed and therein enable the person to reach maximum communication function, work goals and overall quality of life.

Ideally, a key working agreement would be established between the clinic and agency so that issues such as referral processes, timing of referrals and feedback can be discussed and processes implemented and reviewed as needed. It is desirable that the contact in the vocational rehabilitation agency has specific experience in working with people with hearing loss.

Individual clinicians in the implant clinic and vocational rehabilitation counsellors/consultants also need to communicate about the individual client's rehabilitation programmes. Staff in both agencies may be used to being the key person involved with the CI recipient's rehabilitation programme and may need to learn to share this role and/or clarify, and negotiate about, who is the 'lead' agency at any one time in the process. It is essential that the programmes at the clinic and vocational rehabilitation agency are complementary and well timed to maximize the use of resources and outcomes achieved for CI recipients. The clinic's staff should also inform vocational rehabilitation staff about the following:

- The person's functional communication abilities and limitations. Any reports need to avoid audiological jargon such as 'closed set' and replace it with descriptions that are functional and useful to staff working on the return-to-work programme with a client.
- Any precautions related to the implant that could affect type of work undertaken.
- Any other issues, e.g. psychological, social, health issues that impact on a person's capacity to work.

At the point where the CI recipient may begin attending job interviews, it follows that he or she should be offered training to handle the interview situation. The vocational rehabilitation staff or a clinician with appropriate experience could carry this out. In our experience, CI recipients benefit by exploring ways to prepare for the interview, e.g. anticipating questions and vocabulary, learning the names of the interviewers beforehand, and making requests of the interviewer to assist speech understanding. Some individuals may find it helpful to role-play the interview situation with the clinician.

As vocational rehabilitation agencies often employ staff with counselling skills, they may offer expertise in psychosocial rehabilitation that can complement what a clinic may offer, e.g. a clinic and vocational rehabilitation agency could potentially collaborate in conducting group programmes that focus on adjustment issues for people with hearing loss.

One of the difficulties often encountered is that deafened people who are managing to stay in the workforce may still be struggling to cope with under-employment and other workplace issues such as lack of accommodation and greater vulnerability to threats of retrenchment. As they are employed, they may not be eligible for government-funded programmes of assistance. If their job is in immediate jeopardy, and the issues are clearly disability related, they may be eligible for some assistance under a government-funded programme. Such options should be explored and you need to become familiar with the types of employment support programmes available in the area where you are practising. If the CI recipient is ineligible for a government-funded programme or you work in countries where such programmes do not exist, CI recipients or clinic staff may still approach a vocational rehabilitation agency who can offer fee-for-service assistance or suggest another suitable private service provider.

Beyond the implant clinic

As was depicted in Figure 9.1, certain factors make up a CI recipient's core rehabilitation programme. These elements include various counselling sessions, medical assessments, implantation, auditory and communication training, vocational referral and support, etc. However, all good things must come to an end, and so too must this intensive stage of intervention. Despite the breadth of interventions offered by an implant clinic, it needs to be kept in mind that implant programmes are not life-to-death services. Further, because resources are limited, the extent of the interventions needs to be tempered. Positioning a programme as 'there for life' promotes dependency among CI recipients on the centre and sets up centres to fail as clinicians because they become expected to fulfil unfulfillable roles. It would be unethical simply to dump CI recipients when their intensive programme of rehabilitation comes to an end. A staged process of disengagement is required. Elsewhere, strategies for achieving the 'stepdown' are described (Hogan, 2001, Chapter 7). The stepdown refers to the process of gradually preparing your clients (and yourself) for disengagement. Clients should be prepared for the stepdown from the outset. This is more easily done by having a poster in your waiting room and/or a brochure as part of your information kit, which clearly defines the stages of your intervention and anticipated appointment frequency.

A staged approach to the intervention enables CI recipients to see that they are progressing through their rehabilitation programme and that their goals are being achieved. The transition through key stages should be recognized and celebrated appropriately in keeping with the style of your centre. These celebrations are otherwise known as rites of passage. Events such as switch-on (hook-up) come with their own levels of excitement and celebration and are self-evident in themselves. Strategies for preparing a client for stepdown from the intense levels of support that they have been receiving to a maintenance level of support are not so apparent. CI recipients need time mentally to prepare themselves for a transition to a lower level of support. This is best achieved in the first instance by indicating to them that they are nearing the end of their intensive programme and that together you must begin to plan for the transition to lower levels of support. It is worthwhile asking CI recipients how they feel about moving on to a higher level of independence, to identify and work to address any concerns that they may have with regard to this transition and to set in place assurances that any ongoing assistance that the centre can realistically offer will be available. However, it is not a time for false promises. You will not be there forever but, most probably, someone will be. A series of sessions will follow on from this initial discussion but, at a defined date in the foreseeable future, the intensive programme will come to an end.

In addition to preparing the CI recipient for the transition, you as the clinician also need to make preparations. You have given this person a great deal of your professional time and perhaps his or her needs have preoccupied your mind in out-of-work hours too. Just as the CI patient needs to let go of the centre, you too need to let go of the patient. A useful way to make this transition is to have a different person on the team to provide the follow-up services and that this person becomes gradually involved in the last few sessions that you have with the CI recipient. In this way he or she experiences continuity while the role you played in the CI recipient's life begins to diminish as he or she recognizes that it is time to move on to a new stage in care.

Part of the letting-go process is achieved by putting in place (or knowing that they are in place) certain on-going supports for the CI recipient. What are these processes? They can be grouped under headings of personal and technical support. Many of the issues for providing personal support are detailed elsewhere (Hogan, 2001, Chapter 7). In essence, periodically CI recipients will need to see someone just for the support, because at your centre they know at least that someone really understands their needs and will give them a supportive ear. In addition, life crises will arise where CI recipients will look to the centre for support, because this is where they have drawn on support previously. A partner might leave the relationship or vice versa or the person might lose his or her job. An infrastructure needs to be put in place to deal with events such as these. This infrastructure needs to be staffed by suitably trained clinical staff (even if they are perhaps situated in another service or in another building).

Peer support staff (working in voluntary or paid roles) also have a role to play here. Clients need to have been introduced to these people and know how to access them. It is unprofessional, unethical and inefficient to have staff skilled in technology management and/or auditory therapies providing ongoing psychotherapeutic counselling or support work. Very few clinicians possess qualifications in both these areas so the functions need to be clearly separated. When they are not separated, CI recipients persistently presented with problems related to their technology when in fact they were just seeking support and often reassurance. Certainly, make occasional time for such individuals to see you briefly in a supportive setting but do not mistake this for therapy or allow it to become therapeutically oriented, such as in the pursuit of the perfect map. One way for this to be managed is that, when CI recipients come in initially, they first see the support person for a de-briefing and then, if needed (and the need is defined and contracted), they see the specific clinician for a very specified task and time – but only if requested and if required. In the event that the person does present for technological assistance and it becomes apparent that he or simply wanted to see the therapist, issues of dependency once again need to be worked through with the counsellor.

A useful strategy for managing the CI recipients' need to see their old therapist is to see them in the common area, to exchange greetings and pleasantries, and then move on with your duties. Regular attendance by clinicians at peer support programmes and social events, as well as regular newsletters, provide clients with the opportunity to stay in touch, without needing to take up several hours of your clinic time.

We trust that the ideas detailed in this chapter enable you to realize that a CI programme involves more than just giving people a functioning device. Psychosocial factors play a significant role in the probable success of your progamme and therefore must be addressed. Moreover, it is evident that a variety of people, resources and strategies are available to you in addressing these needs so that your intervention may be complete. By complete we mean that the clients can get on with their lives in the manner they envisaged when they engaged your programme, or as near to it as was practically planned for by them in consultation with you. The careful implementation of the strategies outlined here will go a long way towards the realization of such goals to the mutual satisfaction of both the clients and you.

References

Code C, Muller D (1992) Code–Muller Protocol: Assessing perceptions of psycho-social brain damage. London: Whurr

Hogan A (2001) Hearing Rehabilitation for Deafened Adults – a psycho-social approach. London: Whurr

Hogan A, Code C (2001) engaging the client in a helping relationship. In: Hogan A (ed.), Hearing Rehabilitation for Deafened Adults – a psycho-social approach. London: Whurr

Chapter 10
Telephone training with a cochlear implant

ELLEN GILES

Many postlingually deafened adults presenting to cochlear implant (CI) centres describe the loss of the ability to use the telephone as one of the most serious and restrictive consequences of the hearing loss. When CI users who attend the psychosocial communication workshops on our programme are asked what they most hoped to gain from the CI, use of the telephone is frequently mentioned. In our technological world where the telephone can connect us with friends and colleagues instantly, anywhere in the world, the desire to use this facility is very strong. The clinician should therefore be prepared to assess the CI user's suitability and readiness for telephone training, work with the CI user to set realistic and achievable goals, and implement appropriate training exercises where necessary. This chapter offers a hierarchical telephone-training programme with exercises from beginners' level through to activities suitable for the more sophisticated telephone user. Guidelines for assessing the most appropriate level of training are described. Additional materials for this chapter have been developed in conjunction with Merril Stewart from the New Zealand Cochlear Implant Programme and Karen Pedley from Queensland Cochlear Implant Centre in Brisbane. The issue of pre-implant counselling for telephone use is discussed in Chapter 2.

Telephone conversation will present few difficulties for an increasing number of CI users, although for others this aspect of daily communication will be fraught with frustration and a fair degree of stress. Some CI users may attempt a telephone conversation soon after switch-on with varying levels of success. For others, whose profound hearing loss has rendered telephone use difficult or even impossible, sometimes for many years, the prospect of picking up the telephone receiver may be a daunting hurdle – a challenge to be overcome at some future date. No other aspect of CI use relies so heavily on the confidence of the CI user – one incidence of failure may deter the CI user from trying the telephone again for weeks or months. A CI user with 5 years of experience with the implant said of using the phone, 'Confidence is everything.' Giles (1994) reported that 81% of CI users reported feeling anxious or hesitant about using the phone with people they did not know.

In broad terms, understanding on the telephone is correlated with audition-alone, open-set, word-in-sentence intelligibility scores. Dorman et al. (1991) reported 85% of patients with the Central Institute for the Deaf (CID) sentence scores over 60% initiate phone calls, whereas only 31% of patients with scores less than 40% initiate calls. Technological developments in speech processing strategies and the trend to implant adults with more residual hearing have led to a steady improvement in the ability of CI users to discriminate speech without visual cues. The increase in the numbers of CI recipients who report some success in telephone use has paralleled this trend. In the late 1980s, clinicians viewed telephone use as a fortuitous outcome for a small number of CI users, whereas today there is an expectation that the majority of postlingually deafened implant recipients are likely to obtain some degree of telephone use. Cohen et al. (1989) reported that 23% of their adult CI users demonstrated a significant degree of telephone communication ability. Summerfield and Marshall (1995) found that approximately 17% of CI users with a multichannel CI could make effective use of the telephone. Mawman et al. (1997) reported that 29% were able to hold interactive conversation and 83% of the adult CI users used the telephone with varying degrees of ease, depending on speaker familiarity.

Indeed, speaker familiarity is the most significant component of success with telephone conversation. Telephone conversation with an unknown speaker is reportedly the most difficult listening situation for a CI user. Only 15% of CI users on the New Zealand Adult CI Programme could converse with an unknown speaker by telephone with ease, and a further 42% reported that it was possible with 'some difficulty', whereas 33% could converse with a familiar speaker easily and a further 40% were able to do this with 'some difficulty' (EC Giles et al., 2001). Dorman et al. (1991) reported that 48% of CI users who answer the phone could understand a telephone conversation with a familiar caller and familiar topic most of the time. Only 5% reported understanding an unfamiliar caller and an unfamiliar topic.

In Nordic countries use of the mobile phone is particularly high. Sorri et al. (2001) reported that most Finnish CI recipients are telephone users (84%) and 44% also use a mobile phone. Increasing numbers of CI recipients worldwide are mobile phone users and, in a survey by I Anderson (2003), up to 50% of CI users were confident to use the mobile phone in an emergency.

The following procedures for telephone training are more detailed than previously described by Giles (1994). The significant contributions of Castle (1980) and Erber (1985) to this field are acknowledged.

Aims of telephone training

Cochlear implant users may start telephone training with a range of problems and experience. Some will not have used the telephone for many years; others may be able to talk on the phone in a very limited way right up until implantation. When hearing deteriorates to the point where frequent breakdowns occur in conversation, factors such as anxiety, fear, embarrassment and even panic can potentially exacerbate the communication problem and affect the attitude of the CI recipient to telephone use. When the caller is unsure how best to help the CI user, the call may contain many false starts and silences. The caller's response to communication difficulty may range from mild annoyance and irritation to impatience and rudeness. Such responses serve only to reinforce the negative feelings of the CI user towards telephone use.

In the structured approach to telephone training advocated here, the therapist aims to provide the CI recipient with positive experience on the telephone in a controlled environment, build the CI user's confidence in the auditory modality through frequent successes, build a repertoire of conversational repair strategies and, finally, increase assertiveness and conversational partner management techniques to put the person back in control of the telephone conversation.

The CI user may not be able to use the phone as easily as hearing people but with practice many postlingually deafened CI recipients can develop enough skill and confidence to make at least some use of the phone.

The process

A telephone-training programme comprises four stages:

1. Assessment
2. Establishing goals
3. Training
4. Evaluation.

Assessment

The purpose of assessment is to (1) identify the problems that arise when the CI user attempts to use the phone at home or at work, (2) identify the patient's goals for successful telephone use and (3) establish an entry level for training. Typical problems include difficulty in manipulating or operating the equipment, difficulty understanding unfamiliar voices and difficulty identifying the caller.

The CI user's level of auditory discrimination without visual cues should be part of the assessment, because this will give an indication of a starting point for training. An assessment guide (see Appendix 12) is provided to assist the therapist in selecting an appropriate entry level of training.

If previous auditory training exercises have shown that the CI user was unable to achieve open-set discrimination, telephone training with this CI user should commence with the basics of telephone use, discrimination of telephone signals and use of the telephone code (see p. 232).

A minimum score of 50% speech discrimination in sentences (auditory alone) is required to achieve good telephone use (Summerfield and Marshall, 1995). At the University College London (UCL) CI Programme, significantly more CI users (59 versus 14) with scores of over 50% on BKB (Bamford–Kowal–Bench) sentences were able to understand an unfamiliar speaker on an unfamiliar topic over the phone compared with CI users who scored less than 50% on the same sentence test (Aleksy, 1999). CI users with open-set discrimination may find the intermediate level exercises of most value.

If the assessment reveals that the CI user has already experienced disappointments with telephone use, counselling is essential to encourage the CI user to persevere. Factors that influence success on the telephone, such as experience with the implant, speaker familiarity and type of equipment used (e.g. direct input versus electromagnetic induction), should be discussed with the CI user. A staged approach, where task difficulty is carefully matched to the CI user's ability, will reduce the possibility of failure and subsequent further loss of confidence.

If the assessment reveals that the CI user has not used the telephone for many years, the 'rituals' or 'etiquette' of telephone conversation, as detailed by Erber (1985), may have been forgotten and some discussion may be helpful.

Telephone conversation is usually more formal in structure than our face-to-face conversations because the two communicators cannot observe one another's facial expressions, gestures or posture. A typical telephone conversation tends to contain a distinct beginning, middle and end. During a conversation numerous predicable events occur: the speakers greet each other and identify themselves, estimate each other's mood or willingness to talk, establish the purpose of the conversation, estimate the time that is available for the conversation, ask the relevant questions, exchange information and conclude the conversation. Many of our conversational patterns have become unconscious and automatic for experienced telephone communicators. For our CI users, however, it is necessary to analyse these aspects of telephone use, so that they understand what is required for a 'normal' conversation, the ways in which their use of the phone is different from the socially accepted turn-taking process, and how they can use this etiquette to advantage in the early stages of telephone practice.

When the assessment suggests that the CI user is unlikely to achieve sufficient discrimination to permit telephone use, or the CI user does not wish to use a conventional telephone, alternatives may be discussed. These include:

- fax
- pagers
- text messaging
- relay telephone services, e.g. Type-Talk
- email.

Establishing goals

To ensure that the CI user works towards goals that are achievable, the discussion should focus on (1) the CI user's desired outcomes with respect to telephone use and (2) whether such outcomes are realistic.

We have found it particularly helpful to use the Client Oriented Scale of Improvement or COSI (Dillon et al., 1997) to establish goals, because it encourages the CI user to identify particular problem areas, rate the current (or preoperative) level of success, discuss specific outcomes (e.g. whether the goal is to communicate essential information with family members or to be able to use the telephone in a business environment) and also to prioritize them. This will also provide an indication of how important telephone use is to the CI user. An example is shown in Appendix 13.

A hierarchy of telephone conversation levels (Figure 10.1) can be used to explain to the CI user the starting point for training and the steps involved to reach the desired outcome. A similar hierarchy was outlined by Binzer et al. (1999).

Preparation for training

The CI user's individual goals and needs will determine the content of the training sessions. As previously stated, self-confidence on the telephone is gained through success. The likelihood of success can be increased through careful preparation of the environment and equipment, by forward planning, and through the use of a communication partner or 'telephone buddy'.

Easiest

CI user positions handset and discriminates telephone signals

CI user makes a call to a recorded message, e.g. an answer-phone

CI user makes a call to a familiar speaker (family or friend)

CI user receives a call from the clinician

CI user makes a call to an unfamiliar speaker

CI user receives a call from a familiar speaker

CI user receives a call from an unfamiliar speaker

CI user uses interactive telephone menus (pre-recorded)

Most difficult

Figure 10.1 Hierarchy of difficulty for telephone use by a cochlear implant (CI) user.

The environment

Adjacent quiet rooms in the clinic with internal telephone lines are an ideal facility for telephone practice. In this arrangement the CI user and therapist make and receive the call from separate rooms. The support person may remain with the CI user to offer guidance and support or observe the therapist. Close proximity of rooms can save time in the early stages when the calls are very short. In a less optimal set-up, the therapist may need to use a more distant telephone or hospital corridor. Where possible the CI user should use the telephone in the quietest setting to minimize distraction and acoustic interference.

The ideal set-up at home would be a second phone that allowed the CI recipient to call a partner or support person within the house. Alternatively, the CI user may make prearranged calls to a 'telephone buddy' (see p. 226), with support from the partner at home to offer immediate feedback.

The equipment

A systematic trial of assistive devices in the early stages of training will enable the CI users to identify any advantages and increase success rate. A trial of direct auditory input from the telephone to the speech processor, such as a telephone adapter, is highly recommended. For some CI systems, the telephone adapter may be part of the 'accessories kit'. Direct signal input enhances the signal quality as well as reducing or eliminating the input from the processor microphone, thereby reducing the audibility of ambient noise. This is essential where the background noise in the training setting cannot be well controlled. In a study by Nakatake and Fujita (1999), the use of a telephone adapter was shown to improve a CI user's score on speech tracking (from 62.4 to 109.3 phrases per 5 minutes) when compared with perception on the same task over the phone without an adapter.

The potential advantage of a telecoil or induction loop should be assessed. In many countries, telephone handsets are fitted with an electromagnetic induction loop. The telephone 'loop' conveys the signal directly to the speech processor telecoil (either in-built or a 'plug-in' telecoil) by electromagnetic induction. CI users using the recently available in-built telecoils have reported good quality sound and, therefore, it is recommended that this system undergoes trials early in telephone training. A 'plug-in' telecoil is placed on or over the earpiece of the handset. Some manufacturers provide a telecoil phone 'positioner' to hold the telecoil in the correct place. Unfortunately mobile phones do not generally have inductive coils fitted, so the advantage of telecoils is restricted to landline phones. Telecoils may not be as effective as a direct auditory input.

Other equipment that is potentially helpful includes amplified telephones, amplified handsets or in-line amplifiers, which give the listener some control over the volume of the incoming signal, and speaker phones, which some CI users find easier to hear and have the advantage of allowing a helper to monitor the phone call and assist with any difficulties. If the CI user perceives an improvement in reception, use of this equipment is encouraged throughout the training sessions, both in the clinic and at home.

Consideration should also be given to the type of telephone that will be used. The CI user and helper should understand that the variable quality of line connection that may be experienced with cordless phones may make them less suitable for providing successful telephone experience than a landline. Many CI users are keen to take advantage of the convenience of mobile telephones or cell phones, and report good sound reception with the latest digital cell phones, often in preference to landline phones. In addition, features such as caller identification, adjustable volume and SMS messaging mean that an increasing number of CI users are able to make use of cell phone technology.

CI recipients who use cell phones are able to do so by positioning the mobile phone against the microphone of their speech processor. Electronic interference does not appear to be problematic, but the therapist should be aware that some users have reported interference as a buzzing noise when the cell phone is held close to the CI headset or speech processor. CI users should be encouraged to try out a range of mobile phones before purchase to identify those that are most compatible with their CI system and provide the best sound quality. One way of minimizing any interference is to use a hands-free kit. Some hands-free headsets have flat foam earpieces that can be held in position over the microphone of the speech processor. Connection cables that permit direct audio input via the hands-free kit to the speech processor are available, and CI manufacturers may advise which cell phones and connection cables are available and known to work well with the CI system. Cell phone manufacturers, CI advocates and CI manufactures provide information via websites and patient newsletters about cables and accessories for connecting cell phones to speech processors (Tearney, 2002).

Forward planning

The following suggestions may increase the likelihood that the CI user will manage phone calls independently:

- Before initiating a telephone call, write down the information to be obtained or the questions to be asked.
- Consider the likely topics of conversation, so that vocabulary and questions can be anticipated.
- Keep a note pad and pen by the telephone, so that information that needs to be remembered can be written down, e.g. a name that is spelled out.

Telephone buddy

Enlisting the help of a 'telephone buddy' enables the CI user to practise telephone skills in the home environment. A buddy might be a relative, a friend or a partner who has a good understanding of the CI user's hearing needs and is able to be flexible, patient, adaptable and a clear communicator. It is beneficial for the buddy to attend the CI user's telephone training sessions with the clinician, in order to gain an insight into what is required.

Training

Prerequisites to successful telephone training

Understanding the limitations of this medium

At an early stage, CI users should be reminded of the limitations of this medium of communication, even for normal-hearing phone users, e.g. some hearing-impaired adults may have used mobile telephones for text messaging only, and may be oblivious to the problems associated with the acoustic signal. A range of factors can reduce understanding of conversation over the phone including:

- Aspects of the speaker's presentation, e.g. rate of utterance, voice level, accent, speaker not talking into the handset.
- The equipment, e.g. poor line connections, battery failure, signal intermittency of mobile phones caused by transmission strength.
- Aspects of the listener's reception, e.g. ambient noise.

The inherent signal degradation, together with the absence of visual cues, mean that it is normal practice to ask for repeats or clarification over the phone, especially if it is something important such as a name or number. Hearing-impaired people are usually reluctant to ask for repeats or clarification because they feel that this draws attention to their hearing deficit. They may have forgotten that even normal hearing people mishear or confuse some speech sounds such as /v/ and /b/, and /f/ and /s/ on the telephone, and sometimes need to request spelling of a word. Being reminded that this is normal even for hearing people may help to alleviate the CI user's sensitivity to using clarification or repair strategies.

Call initiation

At the start of training, the CI user should initiate all of the calls, even in the clinic. By being in control of the phone call, the CI user can manipulate the topic, the flow of conversation and the length of the call. Initially, the CI user asks for the person he or she wishes to speak to, confirms the speaker's identity, discusses the reason for calling and then terminates the call.

Short call length

Initial practice calls should be kept short. Short calls have less opportunity for communication breakdown, and will thus be perceived as successful by the CI user.

This perception is an important aspect of managing telephone conversations. As the CI user develops a repertoire of repair strategies (see p. 236), call length can be increased with less risk of failure.

Pacing the training

Most CI users find telephone training stressful and tiring. If too many tasks are attempted in one session, the CI user may become tired and fail with the last (and often the most challenging) item. When telephone training is organized into manageable steps, skills, confidence and motivation are increased. There is much to be said for 'stopping while you are ahead', and the therapist should use their experience to identify an appropriate finishing point where the CI user has achieved a task successfully. The motivation generated from successful outcomes is then carried through to home practice and the next training session.

For beginners (an adult returning to telephone use after a long period of non-use, or for a CI user who is not confident in telephone handling skills), positioning of the telephone receiver and discrimination of telephone tones (see below) may be sufficient for a first lesson. In some cases this may be too much to undertake in one session.

Home practice

The CI user should be encouraged to repeat all the tasks again at home using their own telephone equipment with their support person. In our experience, frequent home practice of short durations is most useful.

Levels of training

Three levels of training are described below. An assessment guide is provided to assist the therapist in establishing the appropriate entry level for training (see Appendix 12). Ensure that the CI user has grasped the ground rules of each level before moving on to the next.

Beginners' level

The therapist should work through the following items with the CI user until competency with each skill is achieved.

Positioning telephone receiver

The position of the telephone receiver at the correct height and angle relative to the microphone of the speech processor enhances reception of the telephone signal. Positioning should be practised so that the CI user can readily find *and maintain* the correct position.

An exercise that involves listening to spoken speech, such as a text-following task, is particularly valuable for practising this skill. The therapist reads a passage to the CI user over the phone, using a slightly slower rate of utterance initially, to allow the CI user time to process the information. The CI user follows the same written passage and is asked to repeat the last word whenever the therapist pauses. This provides a check that the CI user has correctly followed the text. Initially, the pauses are made at natural breaks, such as at the end of a sentence or phrase. As the CI user gains confidence, pauses at less predictable places in the text and increasing the rate of speech make the task more challenging.

Discrimination of telephone tones

The ability to identify and distinguish between the signals in Figure 10.2 on the telephone is essential for all levels of telephone use. Using a visual guide, such as the one in Figure 10.2 illustrating the British-style tones, the therapist assists the CI user to identify each of these signals over the phone. You may need to adapt this diagram for the phone system in your country. Once all are readily identified, the CI user may practise discriminating between them.

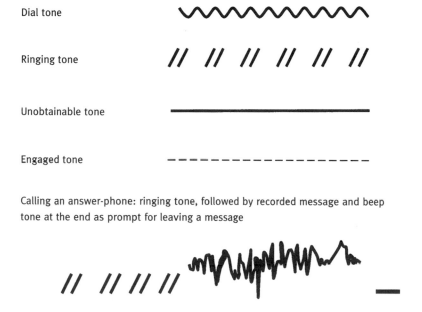

Figure 10.2 Visual guide for training with telephone tones. (Revised version of those found in Castle (1980) and Plant (1984).)

Listening tasks in the clinic

1. Call the answer-phone and leave a short message. (The therapist should ensure that the phone is not answered by another party.)
2. Ask the CI user to count how many times the telephone rings before the answer-phone starts (note that this is subject to individual machine settings).

3. The CI user calls the therapist or telephone buddy at the clinic. Prepared (scripted) responses are available for both parties. This helps the CI user to identify the start of the message. As a first 'conversation' over the phone, all that the CI user may be required to do is respond to the speaker and then 'sign off' and put the phone down.

The response message may be something brief such as:

Therapist:	'Hello, this is [name 1] speaking. How are you? '
CI user:	'Hello, it's [name 2] here. Is that you [name 1]? '
Therapist:	'Yes, it's [name 1] here. Nice to speak to you on the phone.'
CI user:	'Nice speaking to you too! Bye for now.'
Therapist:	'Goodbye.'

This may be practised several times to ensure that the CI user is able to position the telephone headset correctly each time. The therapist should not underestimate the stressful nature of this exercise for some CI users. The therapist should provide plenty of encouragement and positive feedback to the CI user at these early stages of telephone use.

Home practice

- Practise the correct position of the telephone receiver. Identify the telephone tones with the phones available at home. Identify which phone provides the best reception.
- Practise connecting up various accessories. Using the telephone tones, identify which accessory provides the best reception.
- Call an answer-phone and identify the longer 'beep', i.e. the point at which the answer-phone starts to record a message. It may help if the helper or telephone buddy writes down the recorded message, so that the CI user can follow it (like the text-following exercise). Call the answer-phone and leave a (prepared) message
- The CI user calls his or her 'telephone buddy'. The assistance of a third party to receive the call (whether a relative or friend) is particularly beneficial because the support person/spouse can stand by at home to assist if necessary. The CI user is required to:
  - wait for the phone to be answered
  - check the identity of the speaker
  - introduce him- or herself
  - conclude the phone call.

Once the CI user is able to discriminate between the telephone tones readily, the therapist should point out that other combinations might also arise, e.g. when erroneously ringing a fax number the caller will perceive a more electronic, high-pitched noise along with a high-pitched whistle.

Hellos and goodbyes

It is worthwhile asking the buddy to prepare a short introduction that the CI user can readily discriminate over the phone. Some CI users rely on the introductory message by the speaker answering the phone (e.g. 'Hello, John here') to enable them to 'tune-into' and familiarize themselves with the speaker's voice. The helper and telephone buddy should understand that the longer the introduction given by the speaker, the better chance the CI use has of adjusting to the speaker's voice.

Home practice

- Create a list of common phrases used for introductions and closing statements, especially those used by family and friends. Examples of openers include: 'Hello, 345971', 'Hello, Keith speaking'
- Examples of sign-offs include: 'OK, see you soon', 'bye for now', 'ciao', 'thanks for calling'
- The CI user may practise different introductions and sign-offs with the helper (on an internal line in the home) or telephone buddy (outside line).

The use of closed-set questions

A closed-set question is one that has a finite set of answers, e.g. 'Are you calling for John or Betty?' as opposed to 'Who would you like to speak to?'. The CI user can use closed-set questions to limit the possible number of words between which to discriminate. The CI user may adopt this strategy to confirm a message or to confirm the identity of the speaker or caller. Many CI users report difficulties with caller identification, because names are frequently short and contextual cues are limited, if they exist at all. Many CI users also report difficulty in identifying the gender of the caller. The speaker and contextual clues provided by correct caller identification are a significant assistance with understanding the message that follows. For this reason, CI users should be encouraged to limit the number of family and friends whom they call in the early stages of training.

Confirmation of the speaker can be achieved with closed-set questions in the following way:

CI user:	'Hello, it's [name 1] here. Is that you [name 2]? '
Therapist:	'Yes, it's [name 2] here. Hello, how are you?'
CI user:	[and so on with the conversation]

Home practice

- Practise discriminating between the starters and sign-offs with a helper
- Practise a scripted conversation with the buddy
- Prepare closed-set questions that only require a 'Yes, OK' or 'No' answer
- Practise the closed-set questions over the phone with the buddy.

Introduction to use of a telephone code

The telephone code might be considered for CI users who have some discrimination of temporal cues, limited spectral discrimination and limited or no open-set speech discrimination. This method has been used by congenitally deaf and congenitally hearing-impaired adults but could apply equally well to postlingually deafened adults with long-duration deafness. With current-day technology (communication systems such as text messaging or SMS and electronic mail), the phone code is unnecessary for some families. However, as the cost of new technology can be prohibitive, there is still a place for this technique.

The code allows such CI users to be able to use the phone in a limited way, e.g. to convey messages to immediate family or friends, in order to enjoy some degree of independence. One CI user with very long duration of deafness (and poor auditory-alone speech discrimination) used the phone code to prompt her family to respond to her fax messages. The CI user would call her brother and ask him if he had the fax machine switched on and if it was convenient for him to respond to her fax straight away. This saved the CI user becoming frustrated by waiting a long time, sometimes days, for her fax messages to be answered.

Two levels of phone-code approach are described.

Method 1

This procedure was described by Erber (1985) and Castle (1980), and requires the CI user to be able to discriminate between two different temporal patterns such as 'Yes, OK' and 'No'. The contrast has been increased for some CI users by extending the short 'no' into the longer 'nooooo'. Any alternative phrases with which the CI user is comfortable may be used, provided that the CI user can easily discriminate between the two patterns. The main disadvantage is that the hearing person's responses are very restricted. This system also requires a degree of initiative and flexibility by the CI user to phrase questions so that they require only a 'Yes, OK' or 'No' answer, and re-phrase the questions when the unexpected happens. It is possible after some practice to incorporate a third category, a polysyllabic message such as 'Can we discuss this another time?'. The longer response is used to prompt the CI user that the message had not been understood. The CI user would require training to know how best to respond in these situations, such as, 'Oh, there's a problem with what I said, would it help if I rephrased my question?'.

The following is an example of a conversation using the telephone code. The CI user initiates the call. When the phone is answered, the CI user identifies him- or herself with a short introductory message. The conversation continues in the form of closed-set questions from the CI user and pattern-coded responses from the speaker:

CI user:	Hi. It's [name 1] here, remember that we need to use the phone code. If the answer to my question is 'yes' please say 'yes, OK', if the answer is no, please just say 'no'. Do you understand?' . . . [wait for response]
Therapist:	Yes, OK
CI user:	Is that you [name 2]? . . . [wait for response]
Therapist:	Yes, OK
CI user:	Would you like to go for a walk?
Therapist:	Yes, OK
CI user:	Would this morning be OK?
Therapist:	No
CI user:	How about this afternoon, say 2 o'clock?
Therapist:	Yes, OK
CI user:	OK, I'll call around at 2 o'clock. See you then. Bye for now.
Therapist:	Yes, OK. [Hangs up the phone]

Method 2

The method described above can be developed to a higher level by use of a look-up table so that the range of responses can be increased. This method is an adaptation of the 'spelling matrix' (McLeod and Guenther, 1977) which employed a 5 × 6 matrix, each cell containing a letter or a prearranged sentence. In the original version, the position in the matrix would be counted out as 1, 2 and 1, 2, 3, 4, for example. However, this method is now rarely used as CI users who can discriminate numbers are likely to be able to anticipate and understand answers to closed-set questions.

The therapist works with the CI user and family to create the list of responses, making use of rhythm and pitch contrasts to aid discrimination. Both the CI user and family have copies of the set by the phone. The responses can be identified in two ways. The responses are numbered, and the telephone partner indicates the response by number, or (if the CI user has reasonable closed-set discrimination) by using a response from the set. As these become familiar, the reference list may be extended. A CI user used the table of responses in Table 10.1 (p. 234) to call a family member before she left work to make arrangements for dinner.

CI user: 'Hi this is Judy. I'm leaving work now, how are you fixed for dinner?'

Table 10.1 Table of responses

No.	Prearranged responses
1	'That's great. I will see you at home'
2	'I am working late. I will see you at home later. Please start preparing dinner'
3	'I need to go to a meeting. Please go to your sister's for dinner'
4	'I am bringing a take away. Please wait for me at home'
5	'I am already at home. See you soon'

Home practice

• Write a short introductory message.
• Practise use of the introductory message, first without the telephone, then over the phone with the telephone buddy.
• Practise conversation with a family member using closed-set questions (i.e. questions that require only a 'yes' or 'no' response). The questions should reflect the typical questions that a CI user may need to ask over the phone.
• Construct scripted short conversations including closed-set questions and practise these conversations over the phone.
• Practise responding appropriately to unexpected answers. This involves considerable flexibility of thinking on the part of the CI user and not all CI users will find this easy.
• Extend use of the phone code to make a prearranged call to another telephone buddy.

Intermediate level

If the CI user can perform points discussed under 'Beginners' level' with ease, he or she can start on intermediate-level training.

Training in the use of topic and contextual clues

This training aims to show the value of contextual clues and limited-response questions in phone conversations. As a precursor to each training session, it is helpful for the CI user to be familiar with the therapist's voice. This can be easily achieved using a short text-following exercise as described on p. 228.

Listening tasks in the clinic

The following are suggestions for listening tasks over the phone.

Topic-related sentences

The materials used include lists of statements or questions on a related topic such as 'pets'. For the initial exercise with questions, the CI user initiates the telephone conversations and asks the questions so that possible responses can be anticipated. Questions may be used where the answers are likely to be known in the first instance. Examples such as 'Questions about your family' or 'Questions about your holiday' can be found in *COMMTRAM* (Plant, 1984). The CI user can initiate the call, the therapist reads the sentence or questions from the list, and the CI user confirms by either repeating the question or statement or responding to the question, whichever format is agreed beforehand. Initially, this may be performed as a closed-set task where the CI user has a copy of the sentences in front of him or her. To extend the difficulty of the task, the CI user is encouraged to cover the questions and only view them if difficulties arise. Finally, the CI user is given only the topic before initiating the phone call.

Closed-set questions with a closed set of responses

An example can be found in the exercise 'Daily Life' in Watcyn-Jones and Howard-Williams (2002), e.g. the CI user may ask 'Do you have coffee for breakfast?' and the therapist is required to respond from a closed set of four responses, ranging from 'yes, always' to 'no, never', such as 'No, I never drink coffee for breakfast'. This exercise can be used as a turn-taking task so that the CI user has the opportunity both to ask questions and to respond to them. The CI user should repeat what he or she has heard each time so that the therapist can confirm a correct response. The exercise can be made more challenging by the therapist asking further questions on the subject, leading into open-set conversations.

Instruction-following tasks

In this exercise the CI user is asked to follow instructions by telephone that relate to a particular context, set of items or situation. The CI user has a visual context clue by the telephone such as a map. The CI user follows instructions from the helper by telephone. The instructions may tell the CI user to follow directions to a location on the map and confirmed by asking the CI user to repeat the instruction or name the building or place (Plant, 1996). Another example would be to ask the CI user to follow instructions about placing a list of household items (closed set) into a cupboard. The CI user has pictures of the items and the empty cupboard in front of him or her on the phone, and asks the therapist where each item should be placed. The listening task can be simplified by the therapist replying with a carrier phrase such as 'Put the [item] on the left/right of the top/bottom shelf' (Watcyn-Jones and Howard-Williams, 2002).

The task difficulty can be increased by using multiple instructions and/or giving instructions that would not be anticipated.

As the CI user becomes successful in these tasks, the therapist can reduce dependence on closed-set material, and extend the questions and statements to be 'less related' and, therefore, more difficult to anticipate. This will naturally lead the CI user to seek clarification. The CI user should be encouraged to make use of the context. However, it is increasingly likely that repair strategies will be required.

Training in the use of repair strategies

The use of closed-set questioning as a strategy for limiting the content and complexity of the reply has been discussed above. At the intermediate training level, more versatile techniques are required to maintain the flow of conversation. As telephone skills increase, so does the complexity of the conversation. CI users at this level rely heavily on context and prediction for successful management of telephone conversations. Changes of topic, unfamiliar vocabulary and the degraded telephone signal all have the potential to disrupt the flow of conversation. In addition, intermediate level users are increasingly likely to have phone calls with speakers outside the circle of family and friends. Such callers may not anticipate the needs of a hearing-impaired person and will appreciate clear directions when communication breaks down. CI users must learn to analyse carefully and respond skilfully to the various difficulties that they may encounter. The difficulties of managing conversation breakdown on the telephone are exacerbated by the lack of non-verbal cues.

Cochlear implant users reported using a number of strategies on the phone when they experienced difficulty understanding a speaker (Mawman et al., 1997). Seventy-eight per cent asked for a repeat, 46% asked for the information to be rephrased, and 23% requested spelling of difficult or key words. Clearly, some strategies are used more commonly than others, but it is the ability of the CI user to use the most *appropriate* strategy at the right time that results in most successful outcome, e.g. when clarification of a name or other proper noun is the issue, spelling strategies are more efficient than repetition. When the CI user has understood most of the sentence, repetition strategies identify the contextual clues already perceived. When repetition of the phrase results in few words being correctly perceived, re-phrasing is the most efficient strategy.

When the CI user does not understand the message it is neither effective nor sufficient to say, 'I do not understand' or 'What did you say?' The CI user must become proficient in the use of the directive strategies as described by Erber (1985) and listed below.

Repetition

Please repeat the question
Please say the last few words again
Please repeat the first [second, last] word
I got the first bit about [subject], but what was the last bit again please?

Clarification

Did you say [2 o'clock]? This usually prompts either a positive 'Yes, I said [2 o'clock]', or negation, 'No, I said [10 o'clock]'.
Either response enables the CI user to verify the message.

Rephrase

Please say that in a different way
Please use a simpler word; I cannot understand that one
Please use a shorter sentence

Spelling strategies

Please spell that word [you may need to prompt use of the alphabet or phonetic code] (see notes below on the phonetic code)
Please use a code word to spell that (i.e. 'S' for sausages)
What is the first [second, last] letter?
Was that 'p' as in porcupine?
Please say the alphabet slowly until you come to the right letter

Strategies with numbers

Please say each number one at a time
Did you say 'sixteen: one-six?'
Please count very slowly until you come to the right number. Start with the first digit

Clarify or modify speech

I am having trouble understanding your speech:

Please talk more slowly
Please talk louder
Please talk softer
Please talk normally
Please talk into the telephone

Such specific requests carefully guide the speaker to present the misunderstood parts again with 'clear speech'. Picheny et al. (1985) detailed the differences in intelligibility of clear and conversational speech, and Schum (1996) showed that talkers could be trained to use clear speech with minimal instruction and practice that would benefit hearing-impaired listeners. Clear speech was detailed as a communication technique for family and friends in an excellent pamphlet produced by Oticon Corporation (1997).

Clear speech is:

- accurate, precise and fully formed
- naturally slower – this happens automatically when attempting to speak more clearly
- naturally louder – the voice level is raised automatically when attempting to speak more clearly
- lively, with a full range of voice inflection and stress on key words
- characterized by distinct phrases, with breaks between all the phrases and sentences.

Remembering to thank the speaker for assisting (in whatever way) will encourage similar behaviours next time he or she calls.

Listening tasks in the clinic

Exercises that will require the CI user to use repair strategies are listed below. The CI user is encouraged to keep a list of the repair strategies by the telephone.

- The therapist selects names and addresses (from the phone book) and asks the CI user to write them down. Clarification and spelling strategies will be required to confirm that the details have been received correctly.
- This can be expanded into a role-play exercise, whereby the therapist asks the CI user to work as a personal assistant to send a letter to a certain name and address and to send it by courier, fax or first-class post, etc.

Use of a phonetic code

A phonetic code may be a useful tool when proper nouns (for which there are no contextual clues) must be spelled over the phone. This code uses a word to identify each letter of the alphabet. This could be the phonetic code as used by the emergency services:

A is for alpha
B is for bravo
C is for Charlie (see Appendix 14).

The advantage with this code is that it has already been tried and tested extensively, the words selected being the least likely to be confused with each other. The disadvantage is that it is not very user-friendly; some of the words are not very easy to remember, thus requiring both the CI user and the helper, and others, to keep a copy of the phonetic code by the phone.

Some CI users may prefer to personalize their phonetic code and use words that are easier to remember. It is usually a good idea to keep to a theme, such as foods, or animals, e.g.

A is for apple
B is for banana
C is for carrot
and so on.

It would be necessary to check that the CI user can distinguish easily between the selection of words, and to replace any words that are not easily perceived.

Home practice

The following home practice is recommended at this stage:

- The CI user makes a daily call to a friend or telephone buddy for a short (say, 2 minutes) 'chat' on an agreed subject. This usually takes the format of discussing what each person has done that day where daily routines would already be well known.
- Once this has been achieved, the difficulty of the task may be extended by increasing the range of subjects discussed.
- The length of time on the phone may be increased to 5 minutes.
- The CI user calls another telephone buddy for a short call, thus increasing the number of telephone helpers.

Receiving calls

Once the CI user is confident to initiate a telephone call, the next level of difficulty would be for the CI user to receive a call from the therapist. It is preferable for CI users to have a helper with them the first few times that they receive a call so that if they do get into difficulties the helper can assist them by:

- helping the CI user to stay calm
- prompting the CI user to use an appropriate repair strategy
- explaining to the caller what the difficulty is and how they can help the

CI user. This type of 'rescuing' should be limited to the initial attempts with this task because, ideally, the CI users will practise these directions for themselves.

- After the call, discussing any 'breakdowns' with CI users, to help analyse how the difficulty arose and what they could say to the speaker the next time they find themselves in the same situation.

As outlined previously, CI users are encouraged to make a habit of 'planning' the conversation: anticipate the topic, consider what information they wish to obtain and, subsequently, the vocabulary, language, statements or questions that may arise. By anticipating what might happen during the conversation, the CI user can consider in advance which strategies to use.

Home practice

- The telephone buddy makes a prearranged call to the CI user on an agreed subject.
- The telephone buddy makes a prearranged call to the CI user commencing on the agreed subject, but then changes the subject. The helper should be prepared to assist the CI user to identify the subject if there are difficulties.
- The CI user attempts to answer a call at home. The therapist should discuss with the CI user all possible options in this situation from the best to the worst scenarios listed below:
  – use a caller-identification system, so that calls are taken only from known speakers
  – attempt to identify the caller and, if possible, take a message
  – tell the caller that someone will call them back later; attempt to obtain a name and telephone number (a caller-identification system would log the number of the incoming call)
  – ask the caller to call back and leave a message on the answer-phone
  – abandon the call.

The last option is clearly not desirable for either the CI user or the caller. The CI user is likely to be left with a sense of failure and despondency, and be wary about answering the phone again. Inability to manage some calls is an inevitable part of the learning process. However, the impact of such calls can be reduced by discussion with the therapist beforehand and the CI user should be counselled about the limits of his or her capabilities. A proactive approach encouraging discussion of each problem call with the therapist, and how a similar call may be tackled in the future, is encouraged, although a diary approach is often useful to help the CI user gauge his or her progress (see Chapter 4 for further details).

Where people get stuck – asking for help and ways of moving on!

Managing a telephone conversation assertively will assist the CI user to be more effective on the telephone. However, not all CI users are able or willing to be assertive and indeed some CI users perceive all telephone difficulties as their own making. It is consequently worthwhile exploring with the CI user why he or she found it difficult to make requests of the caller.

Some common responses are:

- The request draws attention to my hearing impairment.
- I feel uncomfortable asking for help.
- It is not worthwhile. Having asked for help once, many CI users felt that the modification they requested, e.g. to speak more slowly, was not maintained by the speaker.

Other points for discussion include:

- Re-visiting the CI user's goals
- Listing the potential benefits of receiving calls from regular callers who have a better understanding of their hearing needs
- Accepting that some individuals will be helpful, whereas others will not
- Changing speech patterns may be maintained by the speaker with some reminders.

Where the CI user requires assertiveness training in all communication contexts, the reader is directed to Chapter 7. Some CI users may be assertive in one-on-one conversation but not transfer this skill to the telephone. Where discussion of assertiveness specifically on the telephone is required, Exercise 9 in Chapter 7, p. 161 and in Appendix 5 is recommended. Where group work is a component of the rehabilitation programme, assertiveness on the telephone may be practised in role-play situations with group support.

Advanced telephone use: two-way conversation

Skills building

The essential skills that are required for the CI user to be competent at this level are a good repertoire of repair strategies and the ability to use them in a natural and confident manner in a variety of situations. Training at this level should include opportunities to extend telephone skills:

- Materials that provide opportunities to use repair strategies
- A range of speakers (range of ages, known and unknown, accented speech)
- Receiving calls (again from known to unknown speakers)
- Trial of different phone systems, e.g. mobile, public phone, where the line connection may not be constant or ideal
- Telephone use in different environments (from quiet to noisy backgrounds).

Suggested exercises at this level:

- Connected discourse tracking (CDT) – using a graded reader.
- Interactive exercises where the CI user is required to make an arrangement or booking, e.g. making an appointment to see the dentist or doctor, or answering an advert in the newspaper, such as 'For sale' or 'Renting a holiday home' (Watcyn-Jones and Howard-Williams, 2002).
- Instruction following exercises such as 'Following instructions' exercise, List 7 in *SYNTREX* (Plant, 1996) which requires fine discrimination of speech phonemes.
- Situations that are relevant to the CI user, e.g. business calls.

Some advanced telephone users may be able to use interactive automated telephone menus. Exercises such as checking a bank account balance, listening to current exchange rates or checking on movies showing locally may be possible. Strategies for making this task easier include:

- Obtaining the menu of prompts first (e.g. from the bank)
- Listening to the menu with the written prompts in front of you and listen to all of the messages
- Asking someone to listen to the prompts and writing them down
- Identifying the option that transfers you to an operator before you begin
- Having any passwords required written down in front of you.

CI users starting at an advanced level are likely to demonstrate good open-set speech discrimination. However, this does not necessarily mean that they also have a good command of repair strategies or the confidence to apply them. The therapist may need to use the exercises and materials from the intermediate level before embarking on the exercises above. At advanced level, training sessions may focus on difficulties that the CI user reports in real-life situations, such as dealing with a lost call or with interruptions when using the phone, or managing at telephone conferences. Practice of these difficult situations is likely to be of most benefit to the CI user.

Home practice

- Making phone calls to a range of speakers (e.g. relatives or friends the CI user has not spoken to for some time)
- Picking up the phone when it rings at home and trying to identify the speaker or taking a message
- Making calls to unknown people
- CDT over the phone with a helper (CI user needs to identify all unknown words before moving on)
- Keeping a diary of 'difficult' phone calls, attempted strategies and problems arising.

Evaluation

The CI user has already identified desired goals and/or needs in the COSI. At the completion of the training sessions the COSI is re-administered to determine whether the CI user feels that goals have been addressed or whether further training is required. Evaluation is particularly important, because it enables the therapist both to gauge the CI user's level of confidence with regard to managing phone calls and to plan other courses of action with them where necessary.

Conclusion

This chapter has explored a range of telephone skills and training methods from beginner's to advanced levels of phone use. The importance of outlining realistic and achievable goals at the start, matched to the CI user's capability, has been discussed. The emphasis has been on increasing confidence through successful experience and developing competence through the application of a hierarchy of exercises and appropriate problem-solving strategies.

References

Aleksy W (1999) Telephone use in multichannel CI users. Presented at the Academic Meeting of British Cochlear Implant Group, Spring 1998, York

Anderson I (2003) Telephone use in cochlear implant users. VII International conference on cochlear implants and related audiological medicine. Warsaw, Poland, 22–24 Nov. 2003

Binzer S, Wayner DS, Abrahamson JE, Tye-Murray N (1999) Audiologic Rehabilitation for Adults with Cochlear Implants: Yes! American Academy of Audiology 11th Annual Convention and Exposition, Miami, Florida, April 1999

Castle DL (1980) Telephone Training for the Deaf. Rochester, NY: National Technical Institute for the Deaf

Cohen NL, Waltzman SB, Shapiro WH (1989) Telephone speech comprehension with use of the Nucleus cochlear implant. Annals of Otology, Rhinology and Laryngology, Supplement 142: 8–11

Dillon H, James A, Ginis J (1997) Client Orientated Scale of Improvement (COSI) and its relationship to several other measures of benefit and satisfaction provided by hearing aids. Journal of American Academy of Audiology 8: 27–43

Dorman MF, Dove H, Parkin J, Zacharchuk S, Dankowski K (1991) Telephone use by CI users fitted with the Ineraid cochlear implant. Ear and Hearing 12: 368–9

Erber NP (1985) Telephone Communication and Hearing Impairment. London: Taylor & Francis

Giles EC (1994) An outline of telephone training procedures at the Manchester Cochlear Implant Centre. In: Hochmair-Desoyer JL, Hochmair ES (eds), Advances in Cochlear Implants. Vienna: Manz, 604–8

Giles EC, Kelly A, Jerram C (2001) Clinical Audit of the New Zealand CI Programme (adults). Internal report to Cochlear Implant Clinical Committee, Feb 2001.

McLeod R, Guenther M (1977) Use of an ordinary telephone by an oral deaf person: A case history. Volta Review 79: 435–42

Mawman DJ, Giles EC, O'Driscoll M, Hamrouge S, Ramsden RT (1997) Telephone use by cochlear implant users in Manchester. Poster presented at the Vth International CI Conference, New York City, 1–3 May 1997

Nakatake IJ, Fujita S (1999) Hearing ability by telephone of CI users with cochlear implants. Otolaryngology – Head and Neck Surgery 121: 802–4

Oticon Corporation (1997) Clear Speech: A communication technique for family and friends. Denmark: Oticon Corporation

Picheny M, Braida L, Durlach N (1985) Speaking clearly for the hard of hearing I: Intelligibility differences between clear and conversational speech. Journal of Speech and Hearing Research 28: 96–103

Plant G (1984) COMMTRAM: A communication training program for profoundly deaf adults. Sydney: National Acoustic Laboratories

Plant G (1996) SYNTREX: Synthetic training exercises for hearing impaired adults, revised edition. Somerville, MA: Hearing Rehabilitation Foundation

Schum DJ (1996) Intelligibility of clear and conversational speech of young and elderly talkers. Journal of American Academy of Audiology 7: 212–18

Sorri MJ, Huttunen KH, Valimaa TT, Karinen PJ, Lopponen HJ (2001) Cochlear Implants and GSM phones. Scandinavian Audiology 30(suppl 52): 54–6

Summerfield AQ, Marshall DH (1995) Cochlear Implantation in the UK 1990–1994. Report by the MRC Institute of Hearing Research on the evaluation of the National Cochlear Implant Programme. London: HMSO, 78–81

Tearney L (2002) Cellular phones and the nucleus cochlear implant. In: CICADA: Australian National Newsletter of the Cochlear Implant Club and Advisory Association. April 2002, 1–3

Watcyn-Jones P, Howard-Williams D (2002) Pair Work 1. Harlow: Penguin English Photocopiables, Pearson Education Ltd

Chapter 11
Practical aspects of cochlear implant use

ELLEN GILES

One of the central themes of this book is the holistic approach to rehabilitation. The best outcomes for each patient can be achieved when appropriate support, counselling, and auditory and communication training are combined with technology and a knowledge and understanding of how to use that technology. It is to the practical aspects of the external equipment that we now turn and it is the clinician's role to ensure that patients are fully informed of all the options available to them.

This chapter looks first at the practical considerations of wearing body-worn (BW) and behind-the-ear (BTE) speech processors. Second, we explore the most used accessories and assistive listening devices (ALDs) available, together with their advantages and disadvantages. ALDs are designed to improve perception of speech or environmental signals in poor acoustic environments. The implant manufacturers provide connection cables for ALDs in the patient's accessory kit. Finally, other practical issues such as mobile phone use and use of binaural devices, captioning and communication cards are discussed.

The first part of this chapter explores the counselling and practical issues when the patient is considering whether a BTE or a body-worn speech processor is more suitable. Factors affecting a patient's choice of implant system have been covered in Chapter 2, but some of the issues discussed below may also be relevant.

Factors affecting choice of speech processor

There is a range of issues that will affect patient choice; the appearance will be a big issue for some, whereas, for others, there may be more practical issues. Some MAPs have higher power requirements than an ear-level device can deliver. The cost saving advantage of rechargeable batteries in BW devices is important to some CI recipients.

Practicalities of wearing a BTE speech processor

Convenience

The majority of adult CI candidates opt for a BTE processor for ease of wearing. Adults who have worn BTE hearing aids generally prefer the convenience of having a hearing system at ear level and wish to avoid the use of long cables (as required with a body-worn processor). Generally, the speech processor of all the CI systems is worn over the ear with an ear hook to secure the speech processor to the ear. Patients using the MED-EL Tempo+ have a range of battery pack options – namely, a straight pack, an angled pack and an activity battery pack, which can be secured to clothing (Figure 11.1). Patients are provided with all battery pack options in their kit so that they can choose the configuration that suits their needs.

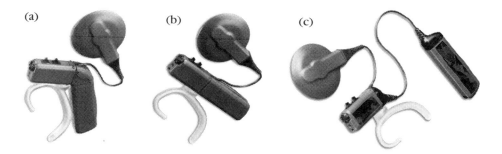

Figure 11.1 The TEMPO+ wearing options: angled, straight and activity battery packs. (Photographs kindly supplied courtesy of MED-EL.)

For new CI users the size, shape and weight of the BTE speech processors may have practical implications such as compatibility with spectacles. The combined 'bulk' of the processor and spectacle frame may be particularly apparent in patients with less room behind the ear, such as when the pinna sits close to the head. Although most CI users do become used to the feel of the device over the ear, potential patient dissatisfaction may be avoided if the patient is able to gain some experience before implantation with the clinic's demonstration device. Patients who have experienced particular difficulties in wearing a BTE hearing aid may opt for a body-worn device once the full implications for comfort are known.

One reported advantage of the BTE processors is that the smaller device does permit 'pillow talk' with partners. For some patients, and perhaps most patients, this may be an important time of the day for personal communication. Patients who find it too difficult or tiring to follow peripheral or group conversation during the day may rely on their communication partner to 'fill in the gaps'. For many patients this 'catch-up' occurs at the end of the day. The BTE processor has the additional advantage over a hearing aid in that there is no feedback with the proximity to the pillow. Thus, this is an important benefit of the implant for some patients.

Dexterity

Clinicians should ensure that patients who favour the BTE device have sufficient dexterity to manipulate the small control switches. The body-worn controls are larger and allow the patient to confirm the settings visually. Patients who cannot manage the BTE controls may compromise their understanding of soft speech, or speech in noisy listening environments, by leaving the processor settings unchanged. In some cases a compromise of appearance, convenience and speech understanding is reached: the patient removes the processor from the ear whenever he or she needs to adjust the volume, sensitivity or choose a more appropriate program. Again, the patients should be aware of all the options and implications of their choice of processor. Interestingly some patients choose to adjust their speech processor settings to suit the acoustic environment whereas others prefer not to make any adjustments. This may correlate with the way these individuals managed their hearing aid systems.

Use of ALDs

Similarly, patients who were regular users of ALDs with their hearing aids are more likely to make frequent use of ALDs with their speech processor. This should be borne in mind when discussing choice of device with the patient. Inputs to the BTE device involve its removal to connect accessories; the inconvenience of temporary loss of sound should be discussed. Patients making daily use of the input socket may notice wear and tear leading to intermittent connection over time. One CI user solved this problem by having a BTE and body-worn processor. For daily use she preferred her BTE processor; however, when answering the phone at her desk, she quickly swapped over to using her body-worn processor, which was already connected via a telephone adaptor to the landline phone, to achieve improved speech perception.

Practicalities of wearing a body-worn speech processor

Securing the processor

The speech processor is the largest and weightiest part of the external equipment and must be secured to avoid possible damage. There are several possibilities: the processor can be clipped on to a waistband, shirt pocket or, particularly in the case of female patients, clipped on to undergarments such as a bra strap. Alternatively, it may be placed in a shirt breast, trouser or skirt pocket. However, patients may quickly discover that wearing the processor in shirt or trouser pockets can be problematic because it tends to slip out at the most unfortunate moments, such as during visits to the bathroom or when bending over. Even if the processor does not actually hit the floor, or worse end up in the toilet bowl, it is likely that the cable may take the weight of the processor with inevitable damage and shortened life. It may also cause an uncomfortable 'tug' on the pinna.

Alternatively, the processor may be placed in a protective pouch that can be worn at the waist or around the neck, usually discreetly underneath the clothes at the neckline. In spite of these options, many female patients, in particular, become frustrated by the limitations to styles of clothing that they can wear because of the speech processor. In particular, in warmer weather or at the beach, the options for processor placement become more restrictive.

Patients whose daily lives involve frequently changing listening situations may consider wearing the processor on the outside of their clothing. This enables them to access the controls, change listening program or plug in an accessory to enhance listening in public places. Thus, one advantage of the body-worn device in this respect is easier access.

Body-worn processor cable

The body-worn processor is connected to the headset or transmitter coil on the head via a cable. The cables are available in a variety of lengths, from 45 to 100 cm, to suit the patient's requirements for wearing the cable. There are a number of options for securing this cable to avoid entanglement (e.g. with door handles, telephone cables, hairbrushes). Wearing the cable under the clothing is one of the best solutions, reducing the likelihood that the microphone or transmitter coil will be pulled off the head, with subsequent temporary loss of sound. However, this does mean that the cable must run up the neck for some of its length and some patients find the cable both irritating and restrictive of their choice of clothing.

Continued snagging of the cable weakens the joints and can reduce the life of the cable. As well as running the cable under clothing, it can be secured on to the collar or underclothes with a spring-loaded clip. Alternatively, a hairclip can be used to hold the cable at the hairline at the back of their head to direct the cable down the back of their shirt or blouse. Some ingenuity is often required to allow patients to wear special occasion clothes such as evening wear. The patient's lifestyle and clothing preferences may thus have some impact on choice of processor style.

Choice of battery pack

Patients with body-worn systems (e.g. Nucleus SPRint) have a choice of battery packs (i.e. one AA battery versus two AA batteries). This apparently small variation can make a difference to the user in terms of overall size and weight of the processor. Patients using a high rate speech processing strategy, such as CIS, might like to ensure that they achieve a full day's battery use with a single rechargeable battery; otherwise a dual battery pack may be a better option. These options are illustrated in Figure 11.2.

(a)   (b)

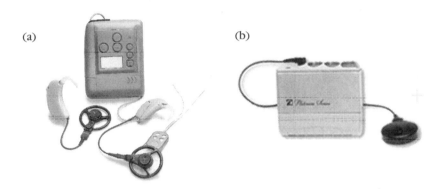

Figure 11.2 (a) The Nucleus SPRint (body-worn) speech processor with detachable battery pack. (b) The Platinum sound processor (body-worn) with rechargeable battery pack by Advanced Bionics. (Photographs kindly supplied courtesy of Cochlear Ltd and Advanced Bionics.)

Rechargeable batteries

The availability and cost of replacement batteries (zinc oxide for Nucleus and MED-EL BTE systems) may be an overriding factor affecting patient choice in some countries. The use of rechargeable AA batteries (provided with the patient kit together with a battery charger) or rechargeable battery pack (the body-worn Platinum sound processor from Advanced Bionics) may be the most cost-effective method of powering a speech processor for some individuals.

Other factors affecting patient choice

Sports and physical activities

Patients who regularly engage in sport or other physical activities at work or for leisure will need to consider both the appropriate style of device and the practicalities of securing both the processor and the cables. A skeletal ear mould may be sufficient to provide a secure anchor for the ear-level microphone of a body-worn system or the BTE device. Some manufacturers supply soft tubing to hold the device more securely around the ear. This significantly reduces the chance of the microphone of the body-worn device or BTE processor falling off the ear. Other patients find that the microphone or BTE processor or transmitting coil can be adequately secured with double–sided tape. For particularly heavy, messy jobs, such as sheep shearing, one adult patient preferred to use a harness on his back to secure his body-worn processor out of the way. Alternatively, users may prefer to remove their body-worn processor if there is a risk of it being damaged.

Cosmesis

Many patients will base their decision for choice (if indeed the clinic is able to offer a choice) of implant system and speech processor on the size, appearance, colour and wearing options of the speech processor. The issue of cosmetics is an important one for many adult and adolescent patients.

Experience suggests that patients appear to polarize into two groups: those for whom cosmesis is secondary to improved hearing ability and those who prefer to wear the processor as discreetly as possible at all costs and therefore opt for the most discreet BTE system. The trend towards 'invisible' aids to hearing, which is largely driven by the desire of the hearing-impaired public to conceal their handicap, is well recognized by those who manufacture and fit hearing aids. In discussing the cosmetic aspects, the clinician should consider the patient's motivation carefully. The implant, like hearing aids, is an aid to hearing and will not enable the patient to conceal his or her hearing disability, especially in noise and group conversation. Where the clinician suspects that the patient is still coming to terms with issues of self-identity and/or acceptance of the loss of hearing, further counselling is recommended. The reader is referred to Chapters 1 and 9 for further discussion of these issues.

Colour options

The CI manufacturers have made colour options available for the BTE systems in response to patient demand. CI manufacturers are aware of this and seek ways to provide patient choice with new colour options and stickers or coloured battery covers to change the 'look' of the processor.

Moisture damage

Ear level microphones (of body-worn and BTE processors) are likely to be damaged by moisture, such as perspiration or rain. For users of BTE speech processors the electronics are also at risk of being damaged and, therefore, higher repair costs are incurred. Moisture damage is a particularly important consideration for users who perspire excessively and for those living in countries with high humidity. The use of a drying agent such as silicon crystals is recommended and should be placed in a bag overnight with the external device. CI manufacturers may have other options, such as a rainjacket to be worn over the BTE processor to protect from excess moisture. Battery performance may also be affected by moisture and humidity, and the use of silver oxide batteries, which are less affected by moisture, may be required.

Making the most of the accessories

The main advantage of ALDs is the improvement in signal-to-noise ratio that they can provide in poor acoustic environments. Using ALDs reduces the effect of distance and noise, both of which result in a loss of audibility of high frequencies, and hence a less intelligible signal. The patient must weigh up the advantage of greater ease of listening against the inconvenience of additional equipment and connection cables. For those patients where the gains are substantial, inconvenience is less likely to be an issue. For other patients, the clinician may encourage greater ALD use by suggesting ways to minimize the drawbacks, e.g. the lead for a microphone may be kept out of the way by passing it under the table in a café. Alternatively, the lead of an accessory, such as the lapel microphone, can be run under clothing and the device passed through a buttonhole and clipped on to the outside clothing. Some patients report that they attach devices in this way before setting out to social occasions. The motivation to use these accessories is likely to be greater in patients with lower levels of tolerance to background noise.

Use of ALDs may also be affected by experience with the implant, e.g. patients who initially report significant benefits from using a direct-input telephone accessory may find that the benefits diminish as their speech comprehension with the device alone improves. At some point, the CI user may find that he or she can achieve sufficient discrimination using the phone without the need to use the telephone accessory.

The most useful accessories

We rarely communicate in quiet places, at ideal distances, one at a time and always facing the listener, so for much of the time communication is a challenge for CI users. The most useful ALDs bring the speaker's voice more directly to the CI user or enhance the quality of other sound sources by removing degrading factors such as distance and extraneous noise.

In the following section the potential uses of each device are outlined. Table 11.1 summarizes the devices together with their advantages and disadvantages.

Lapel microphone

This comprises a small microphone attached to the processor via a cable. It is lightweight, relatively unobtrusive and particularly effective in enhancing the speaker's voice relative to the noise. It works best when placed approximately 10 cm from the speaker's mouth. In our experience it is the most frequently used ALD.

It is particularly helpful in cafés, restaurants and social situations with large groups. It may be worn on the lapel area by the CI recipient or communication partner, or passed 'interview style' from speaker to speaker in a small group or meeting. At dinner parties or weddings it can be passed under the table to improve understanding of speakers at the other end of the table. Patients have also described how they attach it to a glass placed in the middle of the table, enabling them to catch more of the conversation. It can be particularly helpful when the CI recipient sits side by side with the communication partner, such as on a bus, train or aeroplane, and particularly in a car. It may also be passed to passengers in the back seat so that the CI user may follow more of the conversation. CI recipients have reported that they are able to follow the radio better over the road noise (as a passenger) by blue-tacking the lapel microphone to the radio speaker.

In addition, the lapel microphone can be used as a 'back-up' microphone when the user suspects that poor or intermittent sound from the device is caused by a faulty headset microphone. This enables the user to stay on air until he or she can get assistance from the clinic. For this reason it should be demonstrated by clinicians for troubleshooting.

Table 11.1 Summary of advantages and disadvantages of accessory devices

Accessory	Advantages	Disadvantages	Uses
Lapel microphone	1. Effectively improves signal-to-noise ratio (SNR) of speaker's voice 2. Easy to use	1. Best SNR obtained by user pointing lapel microphone towards the speaker 2. Obvious use of equipment; cable must be attached and microphone fixed to lapel or other position 3. Cable may get in the way	Groups Meetings Cafés Restaurants Travel side-by-side (e.g. in a car, train, plane) Rear-seat car passengers Use as substitute for faulty processor microphone
Personal audio cable	1. Direct audio connection provides improved quality of sound for cochlear implant (CI) user 2. Can be used with a range of battery-powered sound sources	1. Movement may be restricted by direct connection to sound source 2. Additional cable	Walkman, Personal CD system Battery-powered radio
HiFi/TV mains cable	1. Direct input reduces effect of distance from TV on signal 2. Integral volume allows balance between signal and environment	1. May cut off signal from TV loudspeaker in some models of TV	TV HiFi Computer Computer games
Direct-input telephone accessory	1. May considerably improve intelligibility 2. Environmental cues still heard	1. Inconvenience if regular phone user 2. Explanation to caller required	Telephone
FM system or cable	1. Effectively improves SNR of speaker's voice 2. Excellent across distance 3. Enables CI user and/or speaker to move about without loss of signal	1. FM equipment expensive and may need careful installation or fitting 2. Requires cooperation of speaker to use transmitter 3. Most FM systems have bulky 'boxes' 4. Transmitter and receiver must be tuned to same frequency channel	Classroom Lecture theatre Golf, biking and other sports involving distances Speaker at a public event or function

The personal audio cable

This cable allows direct audio input from battery-operated sound sources such as a Walkman or personal radio. This might be particularly helpful for home listening practice to cassette tapes or music. Other CI users have reported a preference to listen to music on a Walkman while out walking or doing household chores. This cable should never be used to connect the speech processor with mains-powered devices.

The TV/HiFi cable

This cable allows direct audio input to the processor from equipment powered by the mains electricity supply including the TV, HiFi, radio and computer. The in-line isolator protects the processor and patient from high voltages. Some TV/HiFi cables have integral volume controls. Distracting noise in the room can be made less intrusive by reducing the sensitivity of the processor microphone. Patients report that spending time finding a balance between the TV cable volume and processor sensitivity considerably improves the sound quality and intelligibility. However, for some models of TV, connecting the cable into the headphone socket of the TV may cut off sound through the TV speakers, preventing other members of the family from hearing the programme. This may be overcome by arranging the connection of an additional audio socket to the TV by an appropriate engineer.

Telephone accessories

Telephone accessories, if correctly used, can make the difference between a patient coping and not coping on the telephone. Patients may begin by holding the telephone receiver so that the sound is directed to the processor microphone. Care should be taken with positioning because this can substantially affect the quality and clarity of the speech signal. The in-built telecoil available in the Nucleus ESPrit 3G speech processors should be tried. Similarly the Clarion II BTE processor has a microphone at the end of the ear hook for facilitating telephone use. These devices are illustrated in Figure 11.3.

Some patients manage well and have no need of additional devices. For those who cannot hear well, or cannot maintain the position, a direct-input telephone device can be demonstrated. While this does mean that the CI user answers each call by asking the caller to wait while the device is hooked up, it is usually well worth the effort. Patients who have experienced a good result with a telephone device are usually sufficiently motivated to try it.

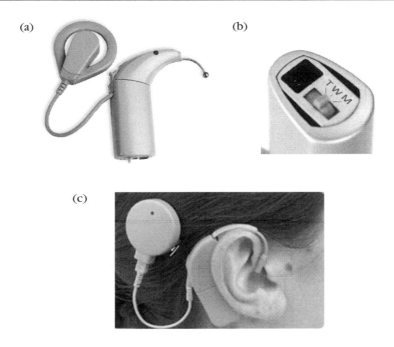

Figure 11.3 (a) Nucleus ESPrit 3G with in-built telecoil. (b) 'T' switch on base of ESPrit 3G. (c) T-mic on Clarion II BTE Microphone positioned at end of the ear hook. The telecoil is in the ear hook. (Photographs kindly supplied courtesy of Cochlear Ltd and Advanced Bionics.)

Alternatively, the accessory kit may include a telecoil or induction loop that is held against the telephone receiver. The signal is transmitted from the induction loop in the telephone handset to the CI telecoil and thence directly to the implant. An accessory is available (Cochlear) to hold the telecoil securely on to the receiver. This telecoil can be used whenever there is a public loop fitted, such as a theatre, cinema or other looped public building. Most public phone boxes are also fitted with telecoil facilities (USA, UK, Australia and NZ). Further information about loop systems is given on p. 258. CI recipients have obtained good results with a speaker telephone. This has the advantage that the support person can listen in and assist the CI user if he or she gets into difficulty. For further information about telephone use and training, the reader is directed to Chapter 10.

Other ALDs

Other ALDs are available either from hearing aid dispensers or from manufacturers of communication aids. Links to numerous manufacturers can be found via the resources section of the website for the Association of Medical Professionals with Hearing Loss (namely www.amphl.org). A discussion of the range and merits of ALDs is comprehensively covered in a presentation 'Demystifying Assistive Listening Devices' at the website of the University of Western Oregon (www.wou.edu/wrocc) under 'training materials' (Davis, 1999).

Assistive listening devices can be organized into the following groups: alerting devices, personal communication systems and systems for public places (loops and infrared systems). Telephone devices have been discussed above. It is recommended that CI centres should have access to a small range of ALDs to demonstrate to patients.

Alerting devices

These include clocks and smoke alarms linked to vibrating pillows or flashing lights, doorbells linked to flashing lights, and cot microphones linked to a loud alarm or flashing light. These may be worthwhile additions to the CI user's accessories, because patients do not usually sleep with the headset/processor in place.

Personal communication systems

FM systems

FM (frequency-modulated) systems must be the ultimate accessory in bringing the speaker's voice to the CI user. It provides a very good signal-to-noise ratio and can be used in a range of listening situations. It is made up of a transmitter, which can be thought of as a small radio station, and a portable receiver, comparable to an FM radio. The system transmits sound using FM radio signals. The FM receiver worn by the CI user requires connection into the speech processor.

The FM system works as follows: the sound source is hooked up to the transmitter. This may be a TV or music input via a connection cable to the auxiliary input of the transmitter. In an educational or training situation, the sound source is more likely to be a person speaking, and the microphone and transmitter should be worn by the speaker, with the placement of the microphone at a comfortable distance from the speaker's mouth, usually 10 cm so that speech can be heard clearly by the receiver. A range of microphones is available and a boom microphone may be more appropriate than a lapel-style microphone for some speakers. The sound source is transmitted as an FM radio wave to the FM receiver which is worn by the CI user. The incoming signal is passed from the FM receiver to the implant via an

FM cable or adapter. The CI user was required to wear the FM receiver as an additional 'box', which made FMs less popular with young people. Recently, the size of some FM receivers (e.g. Phonak Microlink™ CI) has been reduced to allow an FM receiver module to be hooked, piggyback, on to the Nucleus SPRint and SPECTRA body-worn processors. In addition, Cochlear have developed an adapter for the ESPrit 3G speech processors to enable users to access more lightweight FM receivers, such as the Phonak Microlink MLx shown in Figure 11.4.

(a)   (b)

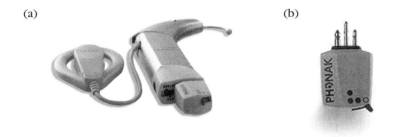

Figure 11.4 (a) Nucleus ESPrit 3G with adapter and Phonak MicroLink MLx attached. (b) Phonak MicroLink MLx (see www.Phonak.com). (Photographs kindly supplied courtesy of Cochlear Ltd and Phonak.)

A range of FM systems (transmitters and receivers) is available and most are compatible with implant systems. Connection cables or patch cords are available from CI manufacturers to enable the CI user to trial alternative FM systems for comparing sound quality and price. CI centres should hold a small stock of FM connection cables, and have access to at least a couple of FM systems. Some countries have a preference for a particular FM system as a result of the encouraged use of this device by the education sector. Similarly, CI manufacturers may recommend an FM system that is known to work well with their CI system.

An FM system may be very useful for group situations where distance is also an issue, such as classrooms, lecture theatres, shopping centres and workplace presentations. The cooperation of the speaker in wearing an FM transmitter may be a significant factor in the successful use of this device. Some deaf–blind CI users have found FM systems useful to keep in touch as their communication partner moves around the home. The FM system may be adjusted to allow input from the processor microphone so that environmental cues (and contributions from classmates, for example) are audible. FM systems can also be used in outdoor activities when the CI user is at some distance from or cannot face the speaker, such as biking or golf.

Personal pagers

Personal communication devices, such as pagers, are available from telecommunication companies, and these enable one-way communication. Pagers typically enable a message to be transmitted to the wearer of the pager as a text message. The caller passes a message via a telephone operator and the CI user is alerted to the message by the pager vibrating. The pager is usually worn in a breast pocket or at the waistband. However, with the advances in mobile phone technology and text messaging (SMS), which enables deaf and hearing-impaired individuals to communicate interactively, the use of pagers has been superseded.

Loop systems and infrared systems in public places

Loop systems can be helpful for listening in an auditorium such as a cinema, theatre, meeting hall or church. Correct installation and function of these systems in public buildings can be an issue because these systems may not always be activated or maintained. Forward planning by the CI user should include a check to ensure that these ALDs work well when required. Also only some of the seats in an auditorium may be looped and this information should be available at the booking office. A test of the strength of the electromagnetic field can provide a useful indication of the best reception in a looped area and to check for 'dead spots'. To use a loop system, the CI user plugs the telecoil accessory directly into their processor, or switches to the 'T' position to activate a built-in telecoil. The telecoil may work better in one polarity than another so this should be practised before it is required.

The use of the infrared system is similar to that described earlier for the FM system, with the sound source connected to the transmitter and the CI users connecting their speech processor to the infrared receiver. A connection cable is required from the infrared receiver into the processor and it is advisable to check the socket connections are compatible, because an adapter may be required. Although loop and infrared systems have the advantage of bringing the sound source directly to the CI user's speech processor, they are prone to interference, e.g. with the infrared device it is essential that there is no obstruction in the path between the transmitter and receiver, otherwise the signal will not be transmitted. Smaller personal loop and infrared systems are also available for use in the home, such as for the TV, but these work well only when the user is not moving around.

Devices for specific needs

Cochlear implant users with specific needs, such as direct input for a stethoscope, should be able to obtain connection cables or patch cords. A supplier of these connection cables can be contacted through the website www.amphl.org

Mobile phones

CI manufacturers may provide, or be able to recommend, a supplier for customized hands-free cable to allow CI users direct audio input to a mobile phone. Customized cables can be used together with an adapter jack to fit specific models of mobile phones. Adapters are available from mobile phone retailers. Use of a hands-free kit reduces radio frequency interference at the head for the CI user. One hands-free system, the Freedom Mach I by HATIS, enables CI users to use the telecoil facility available in some BTE speech processors to pick up sound, hence cutting out background noise.

Alternatively, some patients find that they can hear well enough using a regular hands-free attachment by holding the earphone against the processor microphone. CI manufacturers should be able to provide details of a range of mobile phones that provide good reception with their CI system. Many mobile phones users (hearing and hearing impaired) prefer the vibration mode as a more discreet method of alerting the user to an incoming call. Text messaging is already widely available, making mobile phones a portable form of communication for CI users.

Captions

Many CI users prefer captioned (subtitled) television to supplement their hearing in order to relax and enjoy broadcast programmes and films. It is possible to purchase televisions with teletext facilities but these are expensive; alternatively, teletext adapters can convert standard televisions to provide the option of subtitles. Most videos are produced with subtitles and a captioning unit can be purchased to enable viewers to get the full benefit of captioning with a standard video recorder/player. Similarly a small range of expensive video recorder/players is available that can record subtitled programmes and play these back, as well as providing the captions for subtitled videos. Although this equipment is not universally available, further information can be sought from specialists at the Royal National Institute for Deaf People in the UK who provide impartial advice via their website (www.rnid.org.uk)

Integrating the ALDs with the rehabilitation programme

The various ALDs have been described and their potential uses discussed. However, unless the accessory kit is explained and demonstrated to the patient in a timely fashion and made relevant to the patient, it is unlikely to be fully used. In Chapters 4–6, a structured approach to auditory training is described. Central to this concept is the importance of tailoring the rehabilitation and intervention to meet the patient's specific goals.

During the switch-on period, the patient is usually preoccupied with making sense of the new sound, handling the processor and integrating the implant into daily life. The CI user should also be given his or her accessory kit around this time and the clinician should demonstrate and explain the accessories and how to connect them so that the patient is aware of possible solutions to future problems. Where a range of accessories is provided in the patient kit, it is recommended that the equipment be demonstrated in the same order as listed in the patient user manual, so that the patient has a good reference point when reviewing the kit at home. At this stage few patients experiment with the accessories, perhaps deterred by additional cables and perceived inconvenience. It is more likely that the patients perceive that the implant alone will enable them to cope with most listening situations at this early stage.

Around the time that the map becomes stable, and once the patient has tried a variety of alternative parameters or strategies to find the 'best' map, which is around 3 months after switch-on, the patient begins to appreciate the limitations of the device better. This period, when the patient perceives no further improvement in speech recognition over time, is sometimes referred to as a plateau. The CI user will appreciate that, in some situations, the device together with communication strategies learned as part of the rehabilitation programme do not overcome the difficulties of some listening situations. It is around this time that many patients become interested in discussing the application of the ALDs.

The clinician must pay careful attention to the specific situations described by the patient as presenting ongoing difficulties. These are the problems that the patient is most motivated to solve, e.g. a patient may resume or begin a programme of education; this patient can be reminded to trial an FM system in the lecture theatre, and possibly record the lectures, playing them back later using the personal audio cable. Obviously the telephone devices become more relevant when the patient is ready to begin telephone training. In our experience, ALD use is more likely to be successful if the patient has the opportunity to use the device in the clinic with the clinician before experimenting at home.

Follow-up after initial fitting

A follow-up discussion is recommended at the patient's next visit to establish whether the specific problems have been addressed by the ALD and to offer further assistance if required.

Use of group sessions

Group sessions can be a successful way to motivate patients to try ALDs. Patients benefit from sharing experiences with other CI recipients and may help individuals accept that the implant alone is not a panacea to all listening environments. Group sessions can be dedicated to a particular situation or device such as the telephone. Some clinics may find it useful to include case examples of ALD use in patient newsletters.

Clinicians may also find group sessions to be an effective use of their time. However, individual patients are likely to require follow-up sessions on a one-on-one basis, especially with respect to commencing telephone training.

Use of a hearing aid in the contralateral ear

Several adult CI users have commented that they are very aware of having a 'dead' ear on their other side, or non-implanted ear, and find that they are disadvantaged in a group situation, such as round the dinner table. This can be particularly embarrassing when the CI recipient, engrossed in conversation from the implanted side, is unaware that someone is attempting to get their attention on their 'dead' side. A small minority of patients also complain about difficulty with localizing sound.

For some patients, the problem of a unilateral input can be partially solved by wearing a hearing aid on the non-implanted ear when there is aidable hearing. The fitting of the hearing aid on the contralateral ear has been discussed in Chapter 3. With the increasing trend towards implanting patients with greater amounts of residual hearing, consideration to aiding the other ear will become more frequent. In cases where the *better* ear has been implanted, and very little aidable hearing remains in the non-implanted ear, the benefits may be small. For such patients, a dual microphone headset (i.e. two microphones, one worn over each ear, with input into one speech processor) may offer advantages in some situations (O'Driscoll et al., 2002).

When to introduce the hearing aid

Experience suggests that there are advantages in discouraging the use of a hearing aid in the non-implanted ear for at least the first few weeks and in some cases up to several months after switch-on, e.g. some adults and adolescents who have continued to rely on the more familiar sound from their hearing aid rather than focusing on the new sound through their CI have failed to make progress with the implant. These individuals have complained of the more high-pitched sound of the CI and as a result have tended to keep the sound of their CI turned down relative to the level of their hearing aid. Subsequent withdrawal of the hearing aid in these cases has led to the more usual progress expected with the CI.

However, a more flexible approach may benefit some patients. Here is one case in point. A patient who had enjoyed the benefits of bilateral hearing aids preoperatively preferred to use the hearing aid together with the CI from the outset because she reported that it gave her improved clarity for speech. This was especially important at work where she reported being unable to manage her position without the hearing aid. In a compromise arrangement, the patient undertook daily auditory training exercises with the implant alone in addition to the intensive auditory training sessions provided at the clinic. As experience with the implant increased, she would try to manage with her CI alone at work, until she became tired or needed additional clarity to manage telephone calls, and then she would return to using both inputs together.

In this way she progressed slowly with her CI, but at some stage, between 3 and 6 months after switch-on, the clarity of sound through her CI seemed to improve rapidly and she moved to wearing the CI and hearing aid together full time, reporting no difficulty in integrating the sounds from the two devices. Although assessment of speech discrimination indicated an excellent outcome with her CI alone she continued to prefer to use both devices together.

Practical advantages and disadvantages to wearing both a hearing aid and an implant

Patients using a hearing aid on the non-implanted ear have reported many advantages. Even with poor discrimination on the hearing-aided side, patients report benefits such as increased environmental awareness, better hearing over distance and greater ease of listening. Tyler et al. (2002) reported binaural advantages for hearing speech in noise and localization for two of three patients using a CI in one ear and hearing aid in the other. Some centres encourage patients to wear an aid on the non-implanted side to maintain stimulation of the auditory pathways. This may have some advantage if this ear is later implanted. One practical advantage is that, if the patient finds him- or herself out of battery power, the CI user still has some auditory input.

The disadvantages of combining implant use with hearing aid use relate to the time and expense of maintaining two devices. Both will need replacement parts, periodic re-tuning and daily care. More batteries are required and each device may need different batteries.

Bilateral CI use

Bilateral cochlear implantation is not yet a routine procedure. There are clinical investigations into the additional benefits of a second implant in comparison with the use of the first implant with a hearing aid, or CROS (contralateral routing of signal) device on the second ear. Results indicate that bilateral implantation offers improved speech perception in noise and sound localization (Mawman et al., 2000; O'Driscoll et al., 2002).

The practical issues of bilateral implants indicate a need for highly motivated users. Apart from the obvious need to maintain and wear two devices, the programming sessions are more time-consuming and complex. Each device is individually mapped, and then loudness and pitch are balanced across the ears.

Lapel badges and communication cards

Some hearing-impaired adults find it useful to wear a lapel badge indicating that they are deaf or have a hearing loss. Badges are available with a range of designs from logos of the ear to a brief instruction to the reader, such as, 'I am hearing impaired, please speak clearly'. Lapel badges can convey a clear message, but in my experience few adults feel comfortable about advertising their hearing loss in this way. Indeed it is difficult to know how successful these badges are in conveying the required message to the communicator. Badges and stickers may be purchased from the shop at www.hearing concern.com

Other projects where communication cards have been used are worthy of a mention. In the UK, for instance, a small plastic card (the size of a credit card) called the Hearing Concern Communication card is available. The use of this card is welcome in shops, banks, railway stations and other public places. The idea is that staff should have received training in the communication needs of hearing-impaired people, so that when a cardholder presents their Communication Card on making a purchase or enquiry, staff should immediately recognize the card and use clear communication. Good communication guidelines are detailed on the reverse of the card, such as:

> Look directly at me. Speak slowly and clearly. Be patient and don't shout. Cut out background noise. Write things down or use gestures.
> Hearing Concern (2003, personal communication with Helpdesk coordinator)

In a project called the Hear, Here Campaign in Australia, a group used 'Calling cards' to provide either positive or negative feedback to the hosts of cafés or restaurants on whether the venue was a good place for communication for a hearing-impaired individual. The cards said either 'Thanks: I can hear here' or 'You can't hear here'. There was room on the card for specific feedback, such as: 'the café was too noisy for communication', or 'this was a good place to communicate, we'll come again' (A Hogan, 2000, personal communication).

Summary

This chapter has covered a range of practical issues to assist the clinician with both pre-implant counselling and post-implant device management. In the holistic approach advocated, the patient is not only shown the advantages of supplementing the basic external equipment with assistive listening devices and a bimodal fitting (if applicable), but is also provided with psychosocial support and training to feel comfortable asserting their communication needs.

References

Davis CD (1999) Demystifying Assistive Listening Devices. Website of the University of Western Oregon (www.wou.edu/nwoc)

Mawman DJ, Ramsden RT, O'Driscoll M, Adams T, Saeed SR (2000) Bilateral cochlear implantation – a case report. Advances in Otorhinolaryngology 57: 360-3

O'Driscoll M, Greenham P, Mawman D et al. (2002) Evaluation of bilaterally implanted adult subjects with the Nucleus 24 Cochlear implant system. Paper presented at the 7th International cochlear Implant Conference, 4-6 September 2002, Manchester, UK

Tyler RS, Parkinson AJ, Wilson BS, Witt S, Preece JP, Noble W (2002) Patients utilizing a hearing aid and a cochlear implant: speech perception and localisation. Ear and Hearing 23: 98-105

Appendixes

Appendix 1

Cochlear implant assessment: questionnaire about hearing loss and hearing aids

Thank you for answering the following questions. Your information will help us in making the correct appointments for your assessment regarding suitability for a cochlear implant. We look forwards to helping you to hear better.

About your hearing loss

1. How long have you been hearing impaired? _____
2. How long have you been profoundly deaf? _____
3. Is your hearing loss stable or deteriorating? _____

If you are able to supply copies of any hearing tests this would be very helpful.

About your hearing aids

4. How old are your current hearing aids?   Left_____ Right _____
   Make and model if known: Left_____ Right _____

5. How long have you worn a hearing   Left_____ Right _____ear?
   aid in the

6. Which centre fitted your current   _____
   hearing aids?

7. When was the last time that your   Left_____ Right _____
   hearing aids were fine-tuned or refitted?

8. Please place a tick beside any of the assistive listening or telephone devices below that you have tried:

   ☐ FM System   ☐ Tactile aid   ☐ Loop system
   ☐ Lapel Microphone   ☐ Headphones for TV   ☐ TTY

   Other _____

   Other _____

About day-to-day conversation

9. Is English your first language?   Yes/No

10. When speaking with family and friends, what do you mostly rely on?
    (please tick all those that apply)

    ☐ Hearing aids   ☐ Lip-reading
    ☐ Pen and paper   ☐ Signing

11. When speaking with people in groups, what helps you to follow the
    conversation?

    ☐ Hearing aids   ☐ Lip-reading
    ☐ Pen and paper   ☐ Signing
    ☐ Partners tell me   ☐ I am not able to follow group conversation

12. Which phrase describes how well you can hear on the telephone most
    of the time?

    ☐ I can usually hear when someone calls whom I do not know
    ☐ I can get the gist of the conversation with most people most of
       the time
    ☐ I can hear only people I know well. I often get confused if they change
       the subject
    ☐ I can hear voices on the phone but cannot understand what people
       are saying
    ☐ I do not use the phone at all

When was the last time you were able to hear on the telephone with ease?

_____

13. For moderate-to-loud alerting sounds such as doorbell, phone ring, hail
    on the roof, cars approaching *with your hearing aids* can you

    ☐ Not hear them at all?
    ☐ Hear them some of the time?

☐ Occasionally hear them?

☐ Hear most of them most of the time?

☐ I can't hear them. I am not currently wearing any hearing aids

14. How would you describe your own voice through your hearing aids?

☐ I can hear it and regulate it quite well

☐ I can't hear it very well. My family often tell me I speak too loud

☐ I can't hear my own voice at all through my hearing aids

☐ I can't hear my own voice. I am not currently wearing any hearing aids.

15. To help us in providing background information about cochlear implants, please tell us what information, if any, you have read, e.g. newspaper articles, books, manufacturer's booklets, websites, etc.

_____

_____

I give my consent for _____ to obtain information from other agencies specifically regarding my hearing aid history (as noted above)

Signature _____ Date: _____

Appendix 2

Cochlear implant assessment: expectations regarding outcome and commitment required for a cochlear implant.

Name ————————— Date ————— Seen by: —————

Speech

1 At switch-on I will be able to hear speech but it is unlikely that I will be able to understand any words
2 It may take as long as 6 months to become used to the new sounds
3 Speech may not sound natural to me
4 All words may not sound clear to me
5 I will be able to tell the difference between some but not all voices
6 Speech may not always be easy for me to understand
7 I will need lots of training to make the best use of the new sound
8 Wearing the speech processor regularly can improve my progress
9 The rhythm of speech will be easier to detect
10 I may not be able to understand all speech without lip-reading
11 Learning to identify all sounds may be difficult
12 My hearing will not become normal even after using the implant for a long time
13 Others will still know I have a hearing problem
14 Everyone who has an implant will not eventually have the same hearing ability – outcomes for each person are individual and different

Environmental sounds

1 At first, I may find sounds loud and annoying
2 I will be able to notice many everyday sounds
3 With practice I may learn to recognize many, but not necessarily all, background sounds
4 The speech processor is very sensitive to background sounds
5 I may have difficulty localizing the direction of sound
6 Background noise will always make hearing and understanding harder

Voice monitoring

1 I will be able to hear my own voice
2 I should be able to control the level of my voice with practice
3 The sound of my voice may improve

Lip-reading

1 Lip-reading will still be a major part of my communication
2 I may need to see someone's face to understand words, especially in the first few weeks after switch-on

3 Lip-reading may become less effort when I become accustomed to hearing speech
4 It may be possible to understand some speech without lip-reading when I have gained more experience with my implant
5 I may not understand people talking on television without lip-reading
6 Lip-reading will be especially important when I am trying to hear in noise

Telephone

1 I will not be able to hear on the telephone right away
2 I may be able to understand some speech over the telephone after training and practice

Music

1 Music may not sound normal to me even after using the implant for some time
2 Although I may hear music, it may not sound pleasant to me
3 I may be able to identify a simple song
4 I may be able to pick out the rhythm but not always the melody of the song

Tinnitus

1 I realize there is a possibility that tinnitus may be present or become worse post-implantation

Education and work

1 My education/work prospects may improve, but not singularly as a result of having an implant

Long-term commitment

1 Having a cochlear implant is a long-term commitment
2 I understand that my speech processor will require regular reprogramming (as outlined in the schedule of appointments) for the rest of my life.
3 My progress will be assessed at regular intervals
4 Auditory training exercises practised with my support person will need to be done regularly to maximize my hearing potential.

The above issues have been explained to me. I understand that these are appropriate expectations and the commitment required to get the most out of my cochlear implant.

Signed by client: _____ Witnessed by: _____

Date: _____

Appendix 3

Cochlear implant assessment: information checklist

Name _____ Date _____ Seen by: _____

✓ when discussed

Operation and hospital stay

1 Implant site shaved
2 Length of operation
3 Extent of operation scar
4 Numbness around scar for some weeks
5 Head bandage (adjust spectacles if required)
6 Slight raised area over internal receiver site
7 Length of hospital stay usually two nights
8 Restrictions on medical treatments and activities, e.g. magnetic resonance imaging (MRI), scuba diving, physical contact sports, such as rugby

Operation risks

1 General surgical and anaesthetic risks – discuss with surgeon
2 Risks to facial nerve
3 Tinnitus may increase
4 Possible temporary balance disturbance
5 Possible temporary change in taste

Switch-on

1 Approximately 4 weeks postop
2 Possible eye or facial twitch on an electrode (electrode may be switched off)
3 Large changes in electrical stimulation (e.g. caused by ongoing otosclerosis) may result in changes in sound perception

Rehabilitation and assessments

1 Switch-on will be over 2 days
2 Ongoing appointments schedule
3 Local rehabilitation support can be offered in addition to CI clinic
4 Assessments at switch-on, 1 month, 3 months, 6 months and 9 months post switch-on. Annual reviews thereafter

Costs

1 Travel and accommodation expenses (where applicable)
2 Cables
3 Repairs/ availability of loaners
4 Insurance
5 Battery costs per month (where applicable)

Outcomes

See expectations form

Research projects

The CI clinic is actively involved in a number of research projects. We see this as an integral and essential part of our programme. Our aims are to improve the greater understanding of the function of the hearing system and to improve our services to our CI users.

You will be invited to participate in research projects, but you are under no obligation to do so. These may involve additional visits.

Any questions?

Signed by client: —————————————— Witnessed by: ——————————————

Date: ——————————————————

Appendix 4

Example of post-implant protocol – for local adults

Switch-on week – usually 2 full days

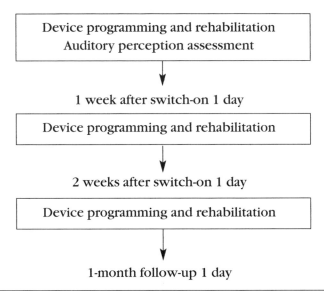

Device programming and rehabilitation
Auditory perception assessment

1 week after switch-on 1 day

Device programming and rehabilitation

2 weeks after switch-on 1 day

Device programming and rehabilitation

1-month follow-up 1 day

Audiology	ORL
Device programming and rehabilitation	Review
Auditory perception assessment	

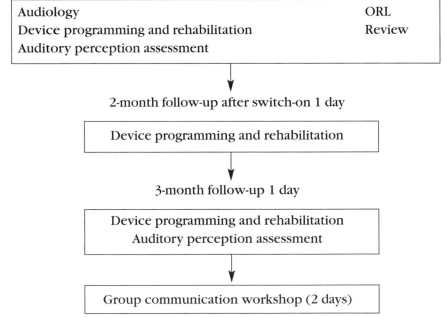

2-month follow-up after switch-on 1 day

Device programming and rehabilitation

3-month follow-up 1 day

Device programming and rehabilitation
Auditory perception assessment

Group communication workshop (2 days)

6-month follow-up 1 day

Device programming and rehabilitation Auditory perception assessment

↓

9-month follow-up 1 day

Device programming and rehabilitation Auditory perception assessment

↓

12-month follow-up 1 day

Audiology Device programming and rehabilitation Auditory perception assessment	ORL Review

↓

18-month follow-up 1 day

Device programming and rehabilitation Auditory perception assessment

↓

2-year follow-up 1 day

Device programming and rehabilitation (as needed) Auditory perception assessment

↓

Yearly follow-ups thereafter – 1 day

Device programming (and rehabilitation as needed) Auditory perception assessment

Appendix 5

Exercises used in Chapter 7

All these exercises are taken from Lind and Dyer (2004). We give permission for them to be photocopied for your own use.

Exercise 1: Tactics for the eye and ear

Flexibility is an important skill in dealing with the many of the problems that may occur in conversation. It can be handy to have a wide range of tactics to help you overcome these problems. Different situations will often need very different solutions. It is best if you can choose those that most directly address the problem, given who you are talking to, and where you are.

Below are some common problems, which may prevent successful communication. List as many different strategies or tactics for overcoming these as you can. You may need to use more than one tactic for some of the problems. Which ones do you feel would solve the problem alone? Which would need to be used in tandem?

The problem

Poor audiovisual cues may arise from:
- sitting too close or too far away from the speaker
- talking in a room that has low lighting
- talking in a room which is visually distracting
- being poorly positioned to follow a conversation happening around you
- talking while the television or radio is on or music is playing
- talking to someone whose speech is quiet or soft
- talking to someone whose speech is too fast
- talking in a group of people where several conversations are going on at once
- talking to someone whose face is in shadow
- talking to someone who is smoking or eating as they speak

Your goal

To be able to see and/or hear the speaker clearly, at a suitable distance, in good constant lighting, without distraction from background noise.

Your strategies

(i.e. what you might do when one or more aspects of this goal are not being met)

1 _____

2 _____

3 _____

4 _____

5 _____

6 _____

7 _____

8 _____

9 _____

10 _____

Adapted and reprinted with permission - **hear**service, VicDeaf. Lind and Dyer (2004)

Exercise 2: Identifying characteristics of the speaker and the message

It is important to be able to identify the commonly occurring behaviours others exhibit in their speech and language. Consider your recent communication partners and try to identify the characteristics of their speech that makes communicating easier or more difficult.

For the characteristics that are not useful consider whether it is possible to change these and how you might tackle the problem.

For example speakers may:
- talk in jargon
- slow down their speech
- turn away while speaking
- repeat turns that you don't hear or understand
- speak while eating or smoking
- speak with an accent that is difficult to follow
- call out from another room
- speak too quickly
- talk about a topic that is unfamiliar to you, and/or
- be unfamiliar to you

Helpful characteristics   **Unhelpful characteristics**

1 _____   1 _____
2 _____   2 _____
3 _____   3 _____
4 _____   4 _____
5 _____   5 _____
6 _____   6 _____
7 _____   7 _____
8 _____   8 _____
9 _____   9 _____
10 _____   10 _____

Lind and Dyer (2004)

Exercise 3: Elements of a conversation

Before any conversation, you can predict a certain amount about with whom you will talk, where you will talk and what you will talk about. We may refer to these three factors as 'the speaker', 'the environment' and 'the message'.

Being able to predict these factors is the first step in helping anticipate potential communication problems and their solutions. Some of the things you can predict may be to your advantage whereas others may be potential hazards that need to be addressed. Choose one or two settings from the list below and under the headings of 'speaker', 'message' and 'environment', make a list of the things that you would expect to encounter. Here are some examples to help you:

The speaker:	quiet voice, clear speech, long moustache, rapid speech, accent
The message:	familiar topic, jargon, short conversation
The environment:	background noise, good lighting, distance from speaker

Here is a list of situations to choose from:

Doctor's waiting room, barbeque, meeting hall, shopping complex, watching television, a bookshop, a situation of your choice

As you consider each of these situations and the factors that will affect your communication you may want to put a '+' beside those that will help your communication, and a '−' beside those that will have an adverse effect.

Setting: _____

Speaker	Message	Environment

Once you have done this you may wish to discuss the possible ways of overcoming the difficulties you have listed.

Here are some guidelines to help you solve these problems:

(i) locate and identify the problems
(ii) take one specific problem at a time
(iii) think about the possible solution(s)
(iv) try this and other approaches out
(v) evaluate the success of the approach

Reprinted with permission from **hear**service, VicDeaf. Lind and Dyer (2004)

Exercise 4: Reactions to communication breakdown

We respond differently to communication problems in different settings. Our responses depend on what problem has occurred, how we feel about it, how the other person feels about it and whether we can quickly find a solution for it.

Describe three situations when your hearing loss affected your communication.

Remember that communication is a two-way process and that communication problems may arise for the other person also.

For each situation, describe:

    (i)   the setting
    (ii) the purpose of the communication
    (iii) your reaction when the difficulty occurred
    (iv) the other person's reaction when the difficulty occurred and
    (v) possible solutions to this situation

If you have trouble thinking of three different situations describe an event at home, at work and in a social setting.

Situation 1

Setting   _____

                        _____

                        _____

Purpose   _____

                        _____

                        _____

Your reaction   _____

                        _____

                        _____

Other's reaction _____

                        _____

                        _____

Possible solutions _____

                        _____

                        _____

Situation 2

Setting   _____

                 _____

                 _____

Purpose   _____

                 _____

                 _____

Your reaction   _____

                 _____

                 _____

Other's reaction _____

                 _____

                 _____

Possible solutions _____

                 _____

                 _____

Situation 3

Setting   _____

                 _____

                 _____

Purpose   _____

                 _____

                 _____

Your reaction   _____

                 _____

                 _____

Other's reaction _____

                 _____

                 _____

Possible solutions _____

                 _____

                 _____

Reprinted with permission from **hear**service, VicDeaf. Lind and Dyer (2004)

Exercise 5: Getting what you want from a conversation

Communication is an art – developing appropriate techniques to compensate for a hearing impairment can be a challenge. Using these tactics in such a way that you achieve your goal in communication is also a challenge. Applying the tactics well relies on developing an appropriate communication style, which is reflected in how you put your message across. Addressing a situation assertively allows you to achieve your goal while recognizing the needs of others. Passive or aggressive behaviours will less effectively allow you to reach your final goal. It is important to be able to distinguish between these behaviour types in any given situation. Below are three responses to the situation outlined. Can you identify which is passive, which is aggressive and which is an assertive response? Which response would you feel most comfortable with?

Situation – at the dentist

Setting the scene:
You have just come out of the dentist's surgery. You want to pay the account and make another appointment. The waiting room is usually quiet but today there is a baby crying in the room. You know from past experience that the dental nurse, who is sitting at a desk, usually looks down and speaks while she is writing. Choose the method you feel you might be happy to use in such a situation.

Response 1:
You walk over to the desk and stand opposite the dental nurse who is sitting down and say: 'The dentist said I need another appointment.' The nurse speaks but you do not hear her clearly, she hands you a card and you leave.

Response 2:
You walk over to the desk pull up a chair and say: 'I need to make another appointment. I would prefer a Monday or a Thursday afternoon, if possible.' The nurse speaks to you but you do not hear her clearly, you ask her to repeat, which she does, you confirm the date and time, and leave.

Response 3:
You walk over to the desk where the nurse is sitting and say: 'I want another appointment. It has to be on a Monday or a Thursday afternoon'. The nurse speaks to you but you do not hear her clearly, so you repeat the same thing. She hands you a card, and you leave.

Having discussed these three examples, you may also like to discuss the following situations. For each one decide what you would think may be the best way you could respond to the situation. Are your responses assertive, passive or aggressive? Why?

Situation 1

You enter a large department store just before Christmas. It is crowded and noisy. You want to buy a travel bag. The shop assistant has a quiet voice.

Situation 2

Your doctor is giving you instructions for your treatment while writing out your prescription. Although it is quiet in the surgery, you are still having trouble hearing him speak.

Situation 3

Someone asks you for directions while you are walking along a busy and noisy road.

In what way is your communication passive, aggressive or assertive?

Exercise 6: Responses to challenging situations

Whenever we find ourselves in a difficult situation, we have the choice of responding to it in very different ways. We can choose not only what we want to say but also how we say it. Both aspects of our communication are equally important.

It is important to find a manner of communicating that recognizes the equality of rights of all the people involved. You can exercise your right to get what you want from the conversation at the same time recognizing the needs of the other person.

Four situations are set out below. For each one write down what you would consider to be a passive, aggressive and assertive response. How do you distinguish between these?

Situation A:

You have been sitting in your dentist's waiting room for nearly an hour past your appointment time. People who have arrived after you have been seen by the dentist ahead of you. The receptionist at the desk seems to be unaware of your lengthy wait. You decide to:

Passive _____

_____

Aggressive _____

_____

Assertive _____

_____

Situation B:

You have ordered lunch for yourself and a friend at one of the outlets in a busy food hall at the local shopping centre. The woman serving you has an accent. She tells you the total cost but you do not hear her. You ask her to repeat which she does but you still do not hear the amount. You say:

Passive _____

_____

Aggressive _____

_____

Assertive _____

_____

Situation C:

You are at a party that is fairly crowded and, as a result, noisy. Conversation is difficult and the person you are speaking to, who is not aware that you have a hearing impairment, is not feeling comfortable about having to repeat so often and is drifting away. You wish to maintain the conversation. You:

Passive   _____

             _____

Aggressive   _____

             _____

Assertive   _____

             _____

Situation D:

You have booked expensive theatre tickets; however, on being seated you find that the seats are not in the part of the theatre you recall booking. You go out to speak to the person in the ticket booth. He says that there is nothing that he can do. You:

Passive   _____

             _____

Aggressive   _____

             _____

Assertive   _____

             _____

Reprinted with permission from **hear**service, VicDeaf. Lind and Dyer (2004)

Exercise 7: Requesting changes in the environment

Once you are aware of the sources of potential conversation difficulty in a particular setting, it is important to feel comfortable requesting changes to alter them, where practical. In the following settings, potential problems have been identified. For each of these, consider what you would do or say to direct others' attention to the problem and attempt to resolve it. In each case keep in mind the difference in aggressive, assertive and passive requests.

1.   You are seated too far from the chairperson at a meeting. You say:

_____

_____

2.   You arrive at a friend's house and the television is on in the room in which you are talking. You say:

_____

_____

3.   When you are seated at dinner, you find that the lamp across the room is shining in your face. You say:

_____

_____

4.   At the doctor's surgery, you cannot hear because of heavy traffic outside the window. You say:

_____

_____

5.   At an evening barbeque, the person to whom you are talking has his or her face in shadow and is standing near the speaker playing music. You say:

_____

_____

6. You are speaking to people across a crowded room, but the distance between you and the volume of the cross talk are too great for you to follow the conversation easily. You say:

_____

_____

7. The bus driver looks away when she tells you what the fare is, you ask her to repeat it, she does, you still do not hear what she has said. You say:

_____

_____

8. You have asked for advice about a product, but the shopkeeper has a very quiet voice. You say:

_____

_____

9. The person you have asked directions from has an unfamiliar accent, and you do not hear any of what he says. You say:

_____

_____

10. The dentist talks to you while standing behind you, and seems to be talking quite quickly. You say:

_____

_____

Exercise 8: Adaptive and maladaptive strategies

The effect of your hearing impairment on conversation will vary from situation to situation. The strategies or tactics that you use to overcome any problems in communication will vary also. Some tactics are useful (adaptive) in overcoming difficulties, whereas other behaviours are unhelpful (maladaptive).

Examples of useful (adaptive) tactics are:

- moving to a quieter spot in the room to talk to someone, and/or
- letting others know that you have a hearing loss.

Examples of unhelpful (maladaptive) behaviours are:

- nodding when you have not heard what has been said and/or
- avoiding social situations you enjoy

Below are listed a number of tactics/behaviours; some are adaptive, some are maladaptive. In the brackets beside each item identify whether you think it is an adaptive (A) strategy or a maladaptive (M) strategy. As you go through them, think about why each item may be useful or not. Which ones do you commonly use? Do they help?

Consider the tactics or behaviours below. Which tactics do you commonly use?

Informing others that you have a hearing loss ☐
Requesting written information when necessary ☐
Directing others to speak more loudly/slowly/clearly ☐
Tuning out, not making an effort to listen ☐
Only doing things that do not involve listening ☐
Reducing background noise ☐
Relying on others to handle difficult listening situations ☐
Avoiding 'non-vital' conversations ☐
Positioning oneself to improve hearing ☐
Interrupting or dominating conversations ☐
Asking for repetition or clarification ☐
Turning up the television or radio without regard for others ☐
Asking for repetition in an abrupt or interruptive manner ☐
Moving to a comfortable distance from the speaker ☐
Expecting others automatically to speak up for you ☐

Getting others to answer the telephone for you   ☐
Maximizing visual cues   ☐
Keeping your hearing loss a secret   ☐
Avoiding asking for repetition or clarification   ☐
Answering questions that you have not understood   ☐
Ensuring that others speak one at a time   ☐
Increasing concentration or attention   ☐

Exercise 9: Asserting yourself on the telephone

When you are having difficulty while on the telephone, there are some aspects of the situation that you may be able to change whereas there will be others that you may not be able to change (e.g. no visual cues). However, an important part of bringing about changes in the conversation that are causing you problems is the ability to request assistance or explain your needs to the person you are speaking to.

It is important in doing this that you are able to present these requests in a polite, non-threatening and assertive manner. This is especially important when they involve the speaker changing his or her way of speaking to help you. Below are set out six difficult situations related to telephone use. Under each of these write out what you would say to the person you are speaking to, to let them know of the difficulty you are having and what needs to be done about it.

Situation 1
You have a poor connection, with a lot of background noise

Situation 2
You find that the woman's voice to which you are listening is too soft for you to hear easily

---

Situation 3
You cannot understand the caller's surname despite asking him or her to repeat it twice.

Situation 4
The man to whom you are speaking is conscious of your hearing loss, and thus speaking very loudly, which is distorting his voice

---

Situation 5
You cannot hear anything of what is being said to you at all

_____

_____

Situation 6
The phone number you have been given is still not clear to you after several repetitions

_____

_____

Reprinted with permission from **hear**service, VicDeaf. Lind and Dyer (2004)

Exercise 10: Effective communication for family and friends

When speaking to a person with a hearing loss, which skills do you feel you demonstrate? Put a tick in the appropriate column.

	Yes	Sometimes	Rarely	No
1. Do you wait to get someone's attention before speaking?				
2. Do you remember to look directly at this person when speaking?				
3. Do you try to imagine what it is like to live with a hearing loss?				
4. Do you move your lips when speaking?				
5. Are you aware that listening with a hearing loss requires enormous concentration, and fatigue often results?				
6. Is your speech clear and at a suitable pace?				
7. Do you remember not to cover your mouth, or turn your back on this person when speaking?				
8. Do you use a few gestures and visual cues (showing objects, writing down names, etc) to assist?				
9. Are you careful about good lighting conditions, so this person can see your face without strain?				
10. Do you repeat words, phrases or sentences without becoming impatient?				

Score (out of 30): 3 points for each 'Yes', 2 points for each 'Sometimes', 1 point for each 'Rarely'

Consider discussing this with the person with the hearing loss.
Do they agree with your self-evaluation?

Reprinted with permission from **hear**service, VicDeaf. Lind and Dyer (2004)

Exercise 11: Effective communication – non-verbal communication

We express our feelings and emotions in many ways – the words we use, our tone of voice, facial expression, gesture and body language, for example. Our non-verbal communication is a very important part of effective communication.

Although we do not often realize it, we 'read' a lot about how a person feels by his or her non-verbal cues. They play an important role in making one feel relaxed and comfortable, uneasy or tense. Different people may be affected in different ways by these non-verbal behaviours.

Under each of the headings below identify examples of that particular behaviour that makes you feel comfortable or uncomfortable. How does a hearing loss affect your use of non-verbal behaviour? How may others react to these changes?

Eye contact

_____

_____

_____

Body posture

_____

_____

_____

Distance/physical contact

_____

_____

_____

Gestures

_____

_____

_____

Facial expressions

Tone of voice/inflection/volume

Reprinted with permission from **hear**service, VicDeaf. Lind and Dyer (2004)

Exercise 12: Problem-solving communication difficulties

An important aspect of communicating with a hearing loss is to anticipate and identify problems and to find creative solutions to these problems. Consider the problems below. Think about the solutions you would implement.

Situation 1

A middle-aged woman who lives alone depends upon the local church for much of her social life. She belongs to a number of committees. She feels her hearing loss makes it difficult for her to 'keep up' on the committees. She is pleased with her cochlear implant but still feels the strain and fatigue at the end of each day. She is feeling increasingly isolated. What can she do?

Situation 2

A businessman is concerned about his hearing loss. He sometimes can't hear on the phone. He finds the meetings he calls in his office noisy and difficult to 'chair'. His desk is opposite the door and staff members often stand in the doorway and talk to him. The noise from the offices beyond intrudes. He has just started using a cochlear implant but has not tried his T-switch. What can he do?

Situation 3

A grandmother enjoys the visits from her grandchildren but they are difficult to hear at times. Their voices are shrill and they often cover their mouths with their hands, they are restless and talk quickly. What can she do?

Appendix 6

What is hearing loss? An audiogram showing the frequency spectrum of familiar sounds

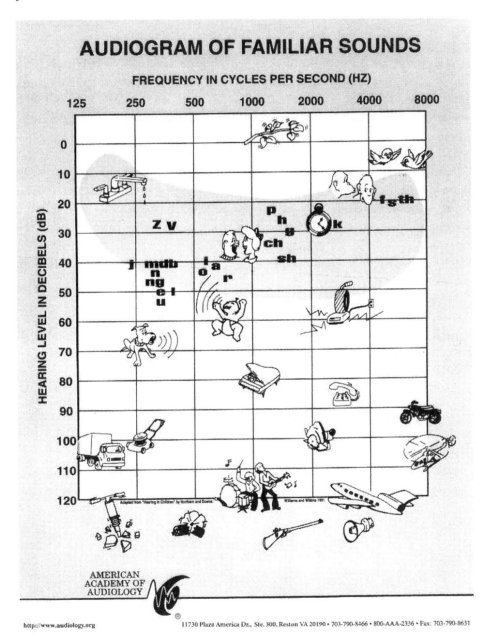

Appendix 7

Sample audiograms to illustrate the effects of hearing loss on speech perception skills

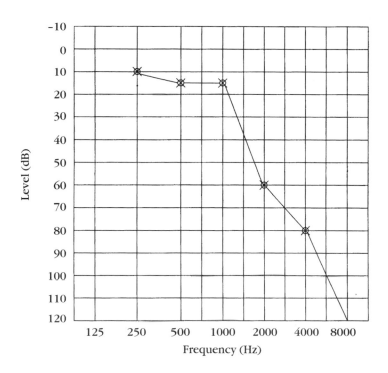

High-frequency sensorineural loss

- Distortions of the incoming signal as high frequency analysis considerably reduced.
- Low-frequency hearing will give acoustic information on laryngeal tones, vowels and nasals. F_2 reduced in /l/ and /I/.
- Friction of /s, z/ not perceived at all (4–8 kHz). Possible difficulty in perceiving friction of f, v, sh, dz, th, ch, especially if low intensity and in discrimination between these fricatives.
- F_2 transitions may be audible to give information on place.

Appendix 7 (contd)

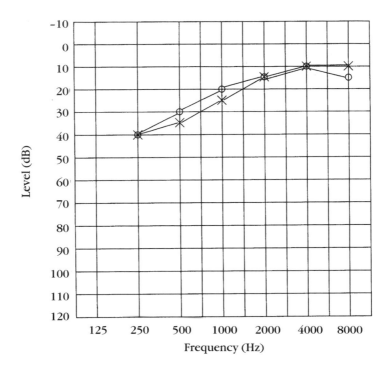

Bilateral low-frequency sensorineural loss

- Hearing in high-frequency range adequate to provide information on place and manner, which is not available from speech reading.
- Acoustic information on lower tones reduced which may influence the discrimination of pitch.
- Little F_1 information leading to difficulties in perceiving vowel quality (close/open) and voicing.
- Possible problems in perceiving /h/.
- For /p, b/ may not perceive place auditorily as energy burst at 600–800 Hz.

Appendix 7 (contd)

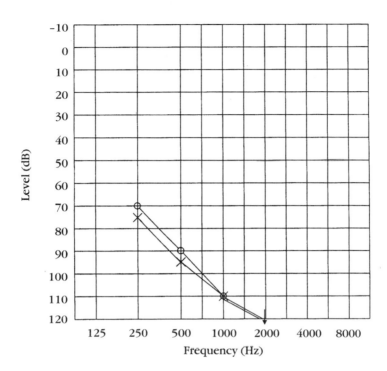

Bilateral sensorineural loss

Possible visual information:
- Facial expression, head movement, etc. may give some indication of rhythm, emphasis, tone moves.
- Consonant placement contrasts: bilabial/labiodental/interdental/postdental.
- Slight rounding of palatoalveolar fricatives in many speakers before close, front vowels.
- Lip positioning of vowels may allow for discrimination between close/ open and rounded/spread depending on phonetic context.

Possible acoustic information:
- Unaided, little auditory information to support speech reading.
- With high-powered aids, might get information on low and mid-frequencies.

- Some information available in the low frequencies, e.g.
  laryngeal tones (may give suprasegmental information)
  vowels, semivowels, liquids (F_1 information)
  no F_2 information so lose information on vowel quality, consonant place
  information from transitions
  nasals distinguished from vowels by low-frequency murmur

Appendix 7 (contd)

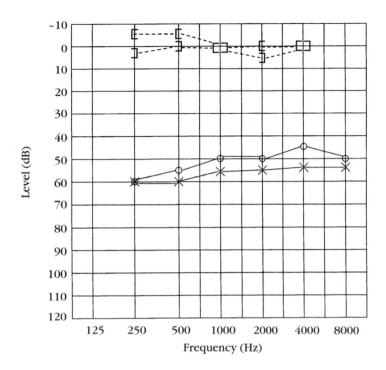

Moderate bilateral conductive loss

- No damage to the inner ear, therefore full frequency analysis without distortion is possible if input is sufficiently loud.
- All speech sounds quieter. Increased need for speech reading in noisy conditions.
- Ability to detect pitch change may be reduced as a result of overall quietness of incoming signal.
- Where intensity decreases, e.g. unstressed syllables, syllables towards the end of a sentence, these may not be heard.
- Friction and affrication may not be perceived as fricatives because of weaker intensity (especially voiced sounds).

Appendix 8

Case history information

Past medical history

_____

_____

Current medical history (including medication, balance and tinnitus)

_____

_____

History of hearing loss

Type of loss (congenital/acquired, sudden/progressive):

Age diagnosed: _____ Age aided: _____

Details of (re)habilitation: _____

_____

Details of hearing aid use: _____

_____

Use of other environmental devices: _____

_____

Audiological information

Dates of recent audiograms: _____

Dates of speech audiometry: _____

Type of device used: _____

Consistency of use: _____

Recommended settings: _____

Audiogram

Language information

First language: ——————————————————————————————

Preferred mode of communication: ——————————————————————

Languages used: —————————— Interpreter details: ——————————

Home: ————————————————————————————————————

Work: ————————————————————————————————————

Socially: ——————————————————————————————————

Speech-reading skills ——————————————————————————

Interests, hobbies, etc.

Appendix 9

Communication skills checklist

	No concerns	Varies with environment	Varies with partner(s)	Assess further/ comments
Speech perception				
Detection				
Discrimination				
Identification				
Comprehension				
Number of syllables				
Speech production				
Phonetic				
Breath support				
Posture/tension				
Voice				
Resonance				
Speech sounds				
Phonological				
Voicing				
Place				
Manner				
Vowels				
Syllables				
Intonation				
Rate of speech				
Stress/rhythm				
Overall intelligibility				
Use of language				

	No concerns	Varies with environment	Varies with partner(s)	Assess further/ cmments
Understanding of language Speech Written Sign				
Expressive language Grammar Semantics				
Interactional skills				
Opening conversations				
Closing conversations				
Maintaining topic: *Own choice* *Other's choice*				
Turn-taking Monitoring partner's reaction				
Use of phatics				
Facial expression				
Body posture				
Gesture				

Appendix 10

Voice profile

Name: _____ Age: _____ Sex: _____ Date: _____ Time of day: _____

1. Quality of voice: normal   breathy   harsh

                                       creaky   whispery   hoarse

2. Loudness: overall   normal   too loud   too quiet

                                         range   restricted   excessive

                                         control   good   limited

3. Pitch: habitual   normal   high   low

                                         range   restricted   excessive

                                         control   good   limited

4. Vocal abuse/irritants:

5. Overall vocal efficiency:

Appendix 11

Taking care of your voice

Alcohol and smoking
1. Some people have a mild allergy to red wine.
2. Alcohol dries the voice. Spirits are particularly bad.
3. Champagne and some white wines (especially sparkling) contain sulphur, which dehydrates.
4. Active and passive smoking dry and irritate the mucosa.
5. Recreational drugs vary in their effects. They may be toxic and constrict breathing. Cocaine irritates the nasal mucosa, leading to vasoconstriction.

Food and drink
1. Acid tea and coffee in large quantities dehydrate.
2. Let hot drinks cool a little before drinking.
3. Drink plenty of water during the day – up to 3 litres for professional voice users ('pee pale!').
4. Fruit juices help to keep the throat moist.
5. If the throat is sore, hourly steam inhalations can help.
6. Some sources recommend a limited amount of dairy products.
7. Acid reflux can irritate the throat. Check the diet and timing of meals.
8. Unless there is an acute infection, avoid medicated lozenges and acid sweets.

Stress and fatigue
1. Learn to relax.
2. Get plenty of sleep.
3. Try to identify what causes anxiety and use strategies to deal with it.
4. Avoid talking over background noise if tired.
5. Rest the voice at the end of a long talkative day.
6. Avoid whispering. It dries and increases tension in the throat.
7. Avoid a 'slumped' posture when tired.
8. Be aware of tightness in the jaw, neck, shoulders and throat. Use chewing and yawning exercises to reduce tension.
9. Avoid gripping the phone while talking. Tension in the arm transfers to the voice.
10. Avoid poor postural habits at work.

Environmental irritants
1. Improve ventilation.
2. Reduce excess heat.
3. Increase humidity – bowls of water near radiators, use of house plants.
4. Drink water
5. Avoid breathing in heavily perfumed air
6. Avoid household and hair sprays
7. Avoid fumes from cleaning products.

Vocal abuse
1. Instead of shouting, screaming or raising the voice try to use another means of getting attention, e.g. whistle, stamping on the floor.
2. Chest infections produce mucus, which needs to be cleared. Huffing rather than persistent throat clearing is kinder to the vocal folds.
3. Swallow, drink chilled water and suck pastilles or chew gum.
4. Do not talk too long on one breath.
5. Delegate tasks needing extensive voice use if possible.

Medical problems
1. Most medication has a drying effect.
2. The voice can be affected by hormonal problems
3. Pain can cause postural changes and tension affecting the voice.

Appendix 12

Assessment guide for telephone training

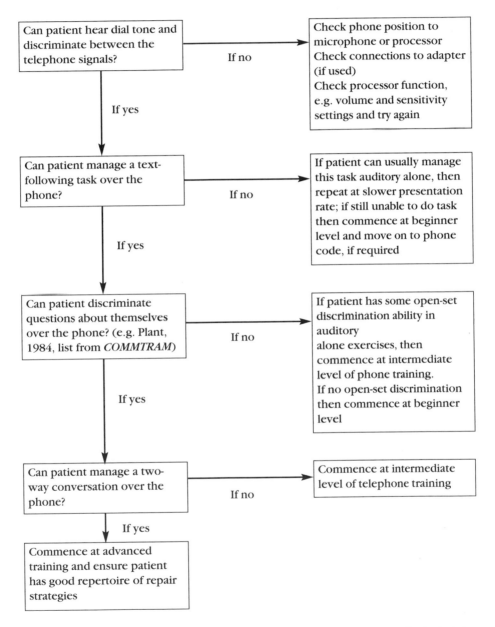

Plant G (1984) COMMTRAM: A communication training program for profoundly deaf adults. Sydney: National Acoustic Laboratories

Appendix 13

Client-oriented scale of improvement (example of goals)

Name: CI user

Date administered: Goals —— 1 —— 2 —— *

Audiologist or therapist: ——

Specific goals

Indicate order of significance

Specific goals	Degree of improvement — Person can hear:					Final ability with cochlear implant — Person can hear:				
	Worse	No difference	Slightly better	Better	Much better	Hardly ever	Occasionally	Half the time	Most of the time	Almost always
1. To be able to hear speech well throughout the call (position of handset to speech processor)										
2. To be able to phone home to let family know if I am going to be late, or if I need a lift										
3. To be able to connect accessories to hear on the phone in noisy situations.										

Key

Use 1 for first administration of COSI improvement and ability.

Use 2 for second administration of COSI improvement and ability.

Source: NAL, Australia

312

Appendix 14

Telephone training – repair strategies

Repetition
Please repeat the question
Please say the last few words again
Please repeat the first [second, last] word
I got the first bit about [subject], but what was the last bit again please.

Clarification
Did you say [2 o'clock]? This usually prompts either a positive 'Yes, I said [2 o'clock]', or negation, 'No, I said [10 o'clock]'. Either response enables the CI user to double-check what has been said.

Spelling strategies
Please spell that word (you may need to prompt use of the alphabet or phonetic code – see notes below on the phonetic code).
Please use a code word to spell that (i.e. 'S' for sausages)
What is the first [second, last] letter?
Was that a 'p' as in porcupine?
Say the alphabet until you come to the right letter

Strategies with numbers
Please say each number one at a time
Did you say, 'sixteen: one-six?'
Please count very slowly until you come to the right number. Start with the first digit.

Rephrase
Please say that in a different way
Please use a simpler word; I cannot understand that one
Please use a shorter sentence

Clarify or modify speech
I am having trouble understanding your speech:

Please talk more slowly
Please talk louder

Please talk softer
Please talk normally
Please talk into the telephone

Phonetic code

A is for Alpha

B is for Bravo

C is for Charlie

D is for Delta

E is for Echo

F is for Foxtrot

G is for Golf

H is for Hotel

I is for Indigo

J is for Juliet

K is for Kilo

L is for Lima

M is for Mike

N is for November

O is for Oscar

P is for Papa

Q is for Quebec

R is for Romeo

S is for Sierra

T is for Tango

U is for Uniform

V is for Victory

W is for Whiskey

X is for X-ray

Y is for Yankee

Z is for Zebra

Index